ESSENTIAL GUIDE ON PRE-DIABETES DIET PLAN TO HELP PEOPLE LOSE WEIGHT

———

Elena Miller

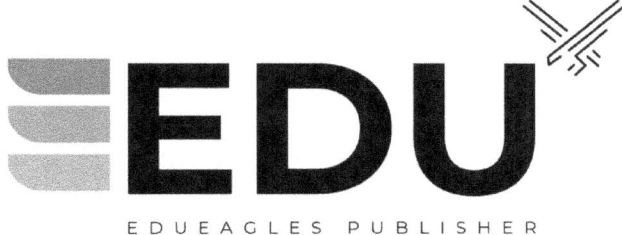

EDUEAGLES PUBLISHER

Table Of Contents

INTRODUCTION

Prediabetes is a lesser known condition than diabetes, but it requires many of the same lifestyle changes as a diabetes diagnosis itself. It basically means that your body has begun to lose the ability to take sugars into body cells for energy. By the time an individual reaches the level of impairment considered to be diabetes, it is pretty serious.

Prediabetes is less severe, but it tells you that you will develop diabetes if you continue on your current lifestyle path. If your doctor has diagnosed you with prediabetes, consider yourself lucky. If you take prediabetes seriously and make changes in your health habits, you will be able to reverse the trend and avoid eventual diabetes. Make the effort now to avoid even bigger complications in the future!

The first step that you should take is to follow your doctor's instructions after he or she has diagnosed you with prediabetes. Depending on how close you are to already having diabetes, you may need to check your blood sugar, take medications, and/or change your eating habits. Follow these instructions to the letter, and ask immediately if there is something that you don't understand.

After instituting the changes ordered by your doctor, there are two more very important things that you need to do in order to avoid developing diabetes. These "miracle" actions are losing weight and getting regular physical activity. Both weight loss and physical activity have been proven to help people reverse the dangerous trend that has begun with prediabetes. Your body can begin to recover its ability to digest and use sugars for energy!

For some people, beginning a weight loss and exercise program can be very intimidating. It doesn't have to be scary, though. Take it one step at a time! If you are not sure what level of exercise you can safely do, ask your doctor before you start. Your physical activity does not have to be strenuous (like running ten miles a day), but it does need to be regular. Walking is a fantastic start for a lot of people. It is relaxing, easy to do anywhere, and

can really burn a lot of calories. If you prefer dancing, swimming, basketball, or any other way to get yourself moving, then that is great. Choose something you enjoy so that it won't be hard to continue with it several times a week.

The physical activity will, of course, help you to lose weight. To help with your weight loss, you may also try to eat smaller portions of the foods you eat throughout the day. Adding in several servings of fruits and vegetables will help as well.

Take the time to take care of yourself now! You can reverse the trend

While it's true that you can't have a "touch of diabetes" as you hear some say, you can certainly have what is referred to as prediabetes. This is a term that has only been in use since 2002. Tommy Thompson, then Health and Human Services Secretary in the G.W

Patients who were given terms such as "impaired fasting glucose" or "impaired glucose tolerance" really didn't understand what they meant.

Other terms that were used such as "a touch of sugar" or "borderline diabetes" were really quite meaningless and people didn't pay any attention to them.

Studies were showing that diet and exercise that resulted in a weight loss of as little as 5-7 percent would actually lower the incidence of type 2 diabetes by up to 58%!

It was felt that a term was needed that would be understood by all. This way, people would know exactly where they stood and where they needed to go with respect to full blown diabetes. People at this stage were at a point where they could make lifestyle changes and avoid the issues surrounding diabetes.

Studies that were being conducted in the early 2000s were showing that most folks who had prediabetes would end up with diabetes in ten years unless they made relatively minor changes in their diet and exercise. It was determined that intervention with prediabetes was critical for three reasons:

By just having blood glucose levels in the prediabetes range, a person had a 50% greater risk of a heart attack or stroke.

The development of type 2 diabetes could be delayed or even prevented by even the smallest of lifestyle changes.

For the vast majority of people, even modest changes would be able to turn back the clock so to speak and return elevated blood glucose levels to normal levels .

WHAT IS PRE-DIABETES?

Most of us have heard plenty about Type 2 Diabetes. It is a serious condition causing abnormal elevations in blood glucose levels. Type 2 Diabetes now affects over 29 million Americans and is costing the healthcare system over $300 billion annually.

The cause of Type 2 Diabetes is multifactorial. A high BMI with an unhealthy diet is often the main culprit, but genetics may play a role as well. Over time, diabetes leads to a host of other diseases, which is where the most considerable health damage is done. These include conditions such as neuropathies, heart disease, stroke, infections, and poor wound healing.

In terms of diagnosis, your doctor will sound the diabetes warning bell if you have an HbA1c above 6.5 and a fasting blood sugar over 125. Treatment often begins with drugs (Metformin is usually the first option) and diet and lifestyle recommendations.

But now more frequently we are hearing about what is termed Pre-Diabetes. Yikes, another type of diabetes? Well, sort of, but not exactly. Pre-diabetes is basically the beginning stages of blood sugar irregularities. It is a critical point where we can catch people before they become full diabetic and in many cases even reverse the progression. It is important that we all get a better understanding of this condition so we can combat the rising rates and healthcare costs of diabetes. To that end let's review the definition of pre-diabetes, the associated health risks, and effective preventative measures.

We already reviewed the diagnostic criteria for diabetes. For pre-diabetes, the ranges are just slightly lower. If your fasting blood sugar is running anywhere from 100-125 and your A1c comes back anywhere from 5.7 to 6.4, you will likely be labeled as pre-diabetic. This puts you at significant risk for diabetes within the next 4-10 years unless steps are taken to return your blood sugar to an ideal range.

This is where I would ask, if you happen to have them on hand or online, to go check your labs. Seriously, go check them! See where your fasting blood glucose is at and determine if you've had a recent A1c. The reason being? Many doctors are not diagnosing pre-diabetes. Studies have shown we have an under-diagnosis problem in this country when it comes to pre-diabetes. I've seen many clients in my office with pre-diabetic numbers and yet no one told them they were pre-diabetic. So yes, go check.

It is so valuable to know this information because pre-diabetes is EASY to treat with diet and lifestyle change. The studies show that diet and lifestyle are the number one

way to reduce blood sugar numbers in pre-diabetic patients. Once you progress to full diabetes the chance of returning to normal blood glucose is much, much harder. NOW is the time to take action and correct .

FOODS TO AVOID FOR A PRE DIABETIC DIET

You might think that going organic if you are diagnosed with pre-diabetes is great. After all, fruits and vegetables are truly some of the best sources of health giving nutrients. Some however, are not very much advisable for consumption by a pre-diabetic individual.

Pre-diabetes is a medical condition which is prior to the full-blown diabetes. It is characterized by a high glucose level. Medical attention is much needed to prevent it from worsening and becoming diabetes. In Pre Diabetic Diet, an individual afflicted with the said condition needs to be very careful on what he or she eats. There are some healthy foods that are not advisable for pre diabetic patients to eat. Simple carbohydrates must be avoided at all times; these produce food cravings and initiate weight gain.

Some examples of simple carbohydrates are:

- ✓ Table sugar and honey
- ✓ Biscuits, cakes, and some puddings
- ✓ Chocolate, candies, and toffee
- ✓ Jam and fudge
- ✓ Mint and boiled sweets
- ✓ Soft drinks and pickles

Fruits made up mostly of simple carbohydrates are:

- ✓ Apples
- ✓ Black berries and blackcurrants
- ✓ Cherries and cranberries

- ✓ Grapefruit and kiwi
- ✓ Melon, oranges and peaches
- ✓ Plum, raspberries and strawberries

Foods with simple carbohydrates are basically health-threatening to a person with a high glucose level. The fruits found above may be consumed by a pre-diabetic individual but at a minimum. Fruits containing more simple carbohydrates do not necessarily create cravings, but they still contain sugar. And sugar is what pre diabetic patients should avoid.

Include in the Pre Diabetic Diet complex carbohydrates instead. They are less likely to produce weight gain and cravings. Complex carbohydrates increase energy level, and

this is very good for health maintenance. They help the body use up most of its stored fats and energy, and are less likely to raise blood sugar

THE DIABETES DIET CURE

Prediabetes and diabetes are the most significant health issues confronting Americans today. In the U.S. today the number of people diagnosed with prediabetes jumped from 57 million in 2008 to 79 million in 2010. Even more ominous, during the same time period, the number diagnosed with full-on diabetes went from 23.6 million to 26 million, the vast majority with Type 2 or adult onset. Put the two numbers together and it accounts for one-third of the U.S. population. Diabetes is a serious issue which can be alleviated by the diabetes diet cure.

Prediabetes means chronically elevated blood sugar levels but not high enough to qualify as diabetes. Prediabetics are "insulin-resistant" as their bodies have become less responsive to insulin, the hormone that keeps blood sugar levels in check. Having prediabetes does not condemn a person to diabetes. Lifestyle changes, including increased exercise and better diet, the diabetes diet cure, will often stave off diabetes or actually reverse full-blown diabetes.

Without the diabetes diet cure, prediabetics will develop diabetes within ten years. Compared with people who have normal blood sugar levels, diabetics are 50% more likely to develop cardiovascular disease and two-thirds of diabetics die of heart attack or stroke. Many prediabetics are completely unaware they are at risk as the condition does not exhibit the typical symptoms of diabetes: heightened thirst, frequent urination, blurry vision and fatigue. Only a blood test can determine for sure if someone is prediabetic.

Who is at risk for prediabetes? Sedentary people and the overweight are most likely to have the condition. Gaining even 11 to 15 pounds for a person of normal weight doubles the risk of developing prediabetes. Of course, larger weight gains mean more risk. This means that at least half the adult population of the U.S. is at risk of developing the disease. The diabetes diet cure can have a major positive impact.

The landmark Diabetes Prevention Program study showed beyond a shadow of a doubt that diabetes diet cure along with moderate exercise can significantly reduce the incidence of prediabetes and diabetes. The 3000 participants in the study were randomly divided into three groups: a placebo group, a group given the diabetes drug metformin and another group receiving intense support for exercise and diabetes diet cure. After three years, the third intensely-counseled group reduced their risk of developing diabetes by 58% compared to those on metformin at only 31%.

What is the diabetes diet cure? It's not that complicated. Eat more fruits and vegetables while avoiding large quantities of meat. Avoid sweets and carbonated beverages. Reduce portion sizes. The goal is to lose even a moderate 5 to 10% of body weight which will produce significant health-protective results. Coupled with moderate exercise, as little as 30 minutes per day, better diet can almost eliminate the condition. The diabetes diet cure alone could completely stop the epidemic of diabetes now threatening this country.

PREDIABETES AND PREVENTION

Prediabetes is a condition in which the blood sugar levels of the body are elevated over a period of time and within a specific range. This condition may be associated with the development of Type 2 diabetes, however ongoing research tends to indicate that there are a lot of strategies that someone with prediabetes can use to prevent or delay the onset of Type 2 diabetes.

Prediabetes can also increase the risk factors for the individual for cardiovascular disease, heart attack and stroke. The condition may also lead to complications with vision and kidney function as the individual ages.

Determining prediabetes factors

Prediabetes factors are measured by your IFG or impaired fasting glucose score and/or the impaired glucose tolerance (IGT). Some individuals may have both IFG and IGT at the same time.

IFG is measured by fasting overnight and then taking the blood glucose test. Individuals with 100-125 milligrams per deciliter are considered to be in the prediabetes range. Approximately 33.8% of the American population age 40-74 will have IFG.

IGT is an oral glucose test that gives a reading of 140-199 milligrams per deciliter after a 2-hour period. Out of the same population of 40-74 year olds 15.4% will have IGT, and 40.1% will have prediabetes.

Can it be controlled?

The good news is that research shows that some lifestyle changes can have a big impact on these factors, and can delay or even prevent the progression to type 2 diabetes. In the Diabetes Prevention program individuals that walked or moderately exercised for 2 _ hours per week, watched what they ate and stayed on any prescribed medication were able to reduce the rate of diabetes by 58% over 3 years. These individuals were all at high risk for prediabetes prior to entering the study.

In addition there are several medications including metformin, and acarbose significantly reduced the rate of type 2 diabetes. The studies showed that the medications were most effective if the participant was between 25-40 years of age and was heavier (60-80 pounds overweight) at the start of the study. Some improvement was also noted in older or less overweight individuals but it was not as marked.

Type 1 diabetes currently has no known methods of prevention. Ongoing studies are attempting to locate the factors that indicate the onset of type 1 diabetes in an effort to be able to introduce prevention programs.

As with all components of diabetes the key to understanding and managing prediabetes is to get the correct diagnosis as quickly as possible. Blood glucose tests should be done if there is a history of diabetes or heart attack or stroke in your family. It is important to also follow through on any recommendations that the doctor may make for further testing. Early diagnosis of prediabetes can allow the physician and the patient to begin to address the issues of weight management, exercise and diet and can lead to the delay or even the prevention of the onset of type 2 diabetes.

PREDIABETES - DIAGNOSIS, TREATMENT AND PREVENTION

Prediabetes, what is it, what are the symptoms, how is it treated, can it be cured? How is it prevented? These questions and more will be treated here in this article.

Prediabetes may be defined as the condition in which not all the symptoms of diabetes is present in a person, but blood sugar level is higher than normal even though not yet high enough to be classified as type 2 diabetes.

In most cases being prior to or being an early stage of diabetes, the characterization of what happens during prediabetes is similar. What is that? Well let's see.

Now ordinarily when food is eaten, the hormone insulin is released by the pancreas to assist the body in the foods processing. Insulin does this by enabling food glucose entry into the body's cells where it will be used for fuel. This action lowers the glucose level in the blood.

However as in diabetes, in a person with prediabetes, the insulin producing organ- the pancreas, either no longer produces insulin, or that person's body cells become resistant to its action or both. Due to this, blood sugar remains at an abnormally high level and this can lead to diabetes with all its attendant complications; heart disease, kidney failure, blindness, amputations, etc.

This latter condition, where a person's body cells become

resistant to the action of insulin is referred to as Impaired Fasting glycemia or Impaired Fasting Glucose (IFG).

Although associated with increased risk of heart disease and insulin resistance, Impaired Fasting glycemia is less of a risk than Impaired Glucose Tolerance (IGT). The difference between the two is that while Impaired Glucose Tolerance emphasizes the insulin resistive aspect of the condition, Impaired Fasting Glucose describes the abnormal blood glucose level of it.

They are related in the sense that a person with a high resistance to insulin, i.e. impaired glucose tolerance is likely to have a higher than normal blood sugar-that is Impaired fasting glucose. However the opposite is not necessarily true - that high IFG correlates to high IGT and in fact it has been found that many patients with impaired fasting glucose have normal responses to a glucose tolerance test.

The criteria for impaired fasting glucose as relates to World Health Organization (WHO) and American Diabetic Association (ADA) standards differ slightly. Whereas the ADA criteria is fasting plasma glucose level from 5.6 mmol/L (100 mg/dL) to 6.9

mmol/L (125 mg/dL), for WHO, the criteria is from 6.1 mmol/l (110 mg/dL) to 6.9 mmol/L (125 MG/dL).

Though Prediabetes does not have any precise signs or symptoms, the prevailing wisdom is that the individual should watch out for symptoms of type 2 diabetes. These include increased thirst and frequent urination, constant hunger, unexplained weight loss, weight gain, flu-like symptoms including weakness and fatigue, slow healing of cuts and or bruises, recurring bladder or vaginal infections, blurred vision, slow healing of cuts or bruises and recurring gum or skin infections.

In addition there are risk factors associated with prediabetes;

being overweight, with a body mass index above 25,

- ✓ being inactive,
- ✓ being aged 45 or older,
- ✓ having a family history of type 2 diabetes,
- ✓ being African-American or a Pacific Islander,
- ✓ being a person having high blood pressure,
- ✓ having a high-density lipoprotein (HDL) or the "good" cholesterol below 35 miligrams per deciliter (mg/dL) (0.9 milimoles per liter, or mmol/L) or a triglyceride (a type of fat in blood) level above 250mg/dL (2.83 mmol/L),
- ✓ having sleep disorders and 9) having a large waist size.

In addition to this if you are a woman - if you have polycystic ovary syndrome - a condition marked by obesity, irregular menstrual periods and excessive hair growth,

having developed gestational diabetes when you were pregnant or gave birth to a baby who weighed more than 9 pounds (4.1 kilograms), then you are at an higher risk.

The American Diabetes Association recommends that people, from the age of 45 (or a person below that age having any of the risk factors mentioned) should consult their doctor for possible blood screening.

The following are tests that a doctor may require you to take to screen for diabetes. The Glycated haemoglobin (A1C) test. This gives a person's average blood sugar level for the past two to three months. A normal A1C is below 5.7 percent whilst that between 5.7 and 6.4 percent is prediabetic;

Fasting blood sugar test. Here, a blood sample is taken and assessed after the individual has gone without food for at least eight hours or overnight. Here, a blood sugar level lower than 100 milligrams per decilitre (mg/dL)-5.6 milimoles per litre

(mmol/L) is normal, between 100 to 125 mg/dL (5.6 to 6.9 mmol/L) is prediabetes or what is sometimes called Impaired Fasting glucose, whilst 126 mg/dL (7.0 mmol/L) or higher is indicative of diabetes.

The Oral Glucose Test may also be recommended although it is rarely used except during pregnancy. Here the individual is given a sugary solution to drink after s/he must have fasted for at least eight hours or overnight. Blood sugar measurement will then be taken after two hours. A blood sugar level less than 140mg/dL (7.8 mmol/L) is normal. From 140 to 199mg/dL (7.8 to 11.0 mmol/L) prediabetic or impaired glucose tolerance (IGT), whilst 200mg/dL (11.1 mmol/L or higher reflects Diabetes.

If the individual does turn out to be prediabetic, then the doctor may require he check that persons HDL cholesterol, A1C, total cholesterol, Low Density Lipoprotein (LDL) cholesterol and triglycerides at least once a year.

So how can Prediabetes be treated?

In this regard, the first necessary thing for adoption is a healthy lifestyle. This will include eating healthy foods. This means a low-calorie, low-fat, high in fiber diet. A diet consisting of more fruits, vegetables and whole grains.

Be more physically active.

A person looking to lower his risk for becoming prediabetic should strive to be physically active. In addition to resistance training like weightlifting, the American Diabetes Association recommends 30 to 60 minutes of moderate physical activity daily.

Lose excess weight. Where you are overweight, losing 5-10 percent of your body weight has been shown to lower the chances of developing type 2 diabetes.

As far as medicine goes, persons considered to be at a high risk of developing diabetes may be required to take the diabetes drug metformin (Glucophage).

With regards to alternative medicine, therapies including chromium, ginseng, cassia cinnamon, glucomannan, prickly pear cactus, coenzyme Q10 and others have indicated promise in the treatment or prevention of type 2 diabetes. However further tests still needs to be made on them. In addition to this, it is also recommended that one consults his/her doctor before engaging alternative therapies so as to enable him give appropriate advice.

Finally, it must be said that prediabetic or not, the adoption of a healthy lifestyle is a boon to good health. In fact it is the key to prevention. As such, irrespective of whether one has a predisposition for developing diabetes or any other disease, the general advice has always been to take it up. That advise remains. It has not changed.

ESCAPE DIABETES - THE 3 KEYS TO BEATING PREDIABETES

If you are one of the 60 million Americans with Prediabetes, here are some encouraging ideas. You have almost a 100% chance to overcome any of the clinical factors that may accompany this label without taking on drop of prescribed medication.

You do however need to overhaul of your diet but this is not the only issue with this syndrome. A wise move to enhance your mental and spiritual level, and practice an energy enhancing exercise can make your symptoms disappear. Developing such mind/ body/ sprit skills will serve you with your overall health now and in your future aging.

Here is the good news part. Right now you body is responding at these 3 levels there is a physical response to a carbohydrate imbalanced diet, a mental response expressed as craving for foods that quickly metabolize into sugar, and a spiritual level that tells you that certain carbohydrates and possibly alcohol is what you need to sustain joy.

This can be corrected by opening awareness to this mind, body, spirit connection to illness and consequently taking action. As a matter of fact any medication taken at this time can put stress on your liver, possible already stressed out from processing too much sugar and alcohol, but not offer any healing.

Real satisfying will come with a determination to naturally take care of your own wellness and a new resolve to not rely on medication to do it for you.

Here is where a wellness practice comes in to boost success to beat Prediabetes. Keep in mind that wellness is a mind, body, spirit process to secure your wholeness. So if you take this route you must deal with the situation as 3 dimensional. What's so good about this is that many have done this before and have been successful and have left a blueprint that you can follow all the way to success.

I am speaking from the voice of experience. When I was in my forties because of my family links to diabetes, I suspected that my light headed symptoms and fainting spells was associated with hypoglycemia or I was becoming pre-diabetic. Since I did not want to be labeled a Prediabetic, IGT - impaired glucose tolerance or hypoglycemic and be stuck in a syndrome of IGT that could proceed to diabetes I decided to nip it in the bud.

My Prediabetes symptoms soon disappeared and that is all it was, revoking symptoms instead of dealing with a disease and all the drama that the clinical world can create around a blood test results. I did not fight! Nor did I march or pay exorbitant medical bills or waste a lot of time in doctors' visits or clinical labs...

But here is what I did do. I decided to become more mentally and spiritually aware of my whole life situation. To quiet my mind at the time, I found a great meditation teacher. I discovered that it is true that meditation releases and enhances the quality of your brain energy and creativity. Once I learned to quiet my mind, Ii was able to creatively focus on this situation without a lot of negative mental chatter. I now had energy to create a lifestyle that helped me to maintain normal blood sugar.

I am now quite well. I get a through yearly check from my wellness physician and for the past 20 years I have had no symptoms of diabetes or blood sugar imbalances.

The first thing that improved was my attitude; I was ready. I became grateful for the opportunity to truly fine tune my diet and looked forward to experiencing the liveliness of balanced energy. Gratitude made it easy for me to accept that some habits had to permanently disappear. Gratitude is a quality of the spirit.

I also found that I was ready to take time and mental, spiritual and physical effort to achieve success...

Another remarkable thing I learned is to trust my own intuition about my well being. This led me to yoga a most balancing energetic process that helped me to appreciate breathing and free oxygen, the molecule that physically runs the energetic process of human bodies.

By now you can get that this is all about developing a healthier lifestyle with a purpose. So regardless of my genetic predisposition, I triumphed.

In the process of cleaning up my lifestyle I became awed by the power of fresh food. Since I was aging so well, I shared these, age without diabetes, recipes in a book. It is now immensely easier for anyone going through this experience to get a handle on the eating part of this process. Every recipe in this book is written with the idea of managing functional hypoglycemia (FH). Because of the amount of processed food available and the introduction of large sugary drinks served with food at fast food places FH is rampant in the US society. So you are not alone. You can also work with a wellness coach to make a smooth transition to a healthier you.

So instead of sulking or OMGing or feeling sorry or angry, all you need to do is change your mind about health, clean up your eating habits and add a few energetic processes like yoga and meditation to your lifestyle. Expect to be amazed at the power

of food, sunshine and movement. You heart will sing because you will ultimately be protecting yourself from heart disease. This is what my mother would call a lagniappe.

And, the pharmaceutical industry will not be so pleased because they will miss out on getting the profits of someone living with disease until the day they die. When it comes to this industry -Building Wellness Kills Profits. I would say that the ball is now in your court.

Celia Westberry, author, speaker and wellness coach has a Master of Science in Cell Biology and is currently CEO of Westberry Wellness Programs. Her goal is to help bring nutritional balance and power to people in search of a happier, healthier more fulfilling life.

She uses this knowledge and experience to design recipes and books to help her clients choose the best food to experience life at the healthiest level. Her book Eat Yourself Younger Effortlessly, the easy way to slow aging, feel, great and look good has glycemic ready recipes to help you take the best eating journey to beat pre-diabetes.

Celia is a competent personal health and wellness coach. As a coach Celia helps clients to open awareness to the awesome, healing power of the mind to promote health and well being.

DIFFERENCES BETWEEN PREDIABETES AND DIABETES

The first thing you need to learn is the difference between prediabetes and diabetes. Knowing what prediabetes and diabetes are, and understanding the similarities and differences between them, makes it easier to find out if you have one of these conditions. Pre-diabetes means that you don't yet have diabetes, but if you do nothing you may develop type 2 diabetes in the future. The biggest worry with prediabetes is an increased risk for heart disease, even if diabetes never develops.

When you have prediabetes you have something called insulin resistance. This means that your body doesn't respond correctly to the insulin your body makes. Your body then has to make more and more insulin to keep your blood sugar levels in the normal range. When you have insulin resistance, other abnormalities of fat and blood pressure occur that can clog your arteries with plaque. So when I talk about treating prediabetes I am talking about preventing both diabetes and heart disease. This condition (and its associated disorder known as the metabolic syndrome, or syndrome X) is very common; more than 44 million Americans have it.

How High Blood Sugar Levels Related to Prediabetes and Diabetes

Diabetes, which is an abnormality of blood sugar levels, is classified by three distinct types. Type 2 is the most common and is the type of diabetes people get if their prediabetes is not treated. Type 1 diabetes is the form of diabetes for which patients must take insulin shots for the rest of their lives. The third type is gestational diabetes, which is a form of type 2 diabetes that can occur during pregnancy. When I treat patients with type 1 and type 2 diabetes, I work with them to bring blood sugar, blood pressure, and cholesterol levels into the normal range. This helps lower their risk for heart disease and stroke (just as in patients with prediabetes) as well as the risk for blindness, kidney failure, and amputation.

When you are first diagnosed with prediabetes or diabetes you need to find health care providers who can give you the education and treatment that you need. Later I will describe how to find helps and who can give it. What is most important to realize right now is that we can do something about prediabetes and diabetes.

Don't Be Desperate if You Have Prediabetes and Diabetes

Having these conditions isn't the death sentence. Think of them instead as an opportunity to take control, to have a longer, healthier life. Many of the diabetes management skills I hope to I can make you (actually anyone) healthier overall. Fixing one part of your health - for instance, increasing the fiber in your diet to help lower blood sugar and cholesterol levels, can also affect another area, such a lowering the risk for colon cancer. Treating diabetes is treating your well-being overall.

How diet relates to prediabetes

There are many factors that increase your risk for prediabetes. Genetics can play a role, especially if diabetes runs in your family. However, lifestyle factors play a larger role in the development of disease. Excess body fat and a sedentary lifestyle are other potential risk factors.

In prediabetes, sugar from food begins to build up in your bloodstream because insulin can't easily move it into your cells.

Eating carbohydrates doesn't cause prediabetes. The amount and type of carbohydrates consumed in a meal is what influences blood sugar. A diet filled with refined and processed carbohydrates that digest quickly can cause higher spikes in blood sugar.

For most people with prediabetes, the body has a difficult time lowering blood sugar levels after meals. Avoiding blood sugar spikes can help.

When you eat more calories than your body needs, they get stored as fat. This can cause you to gain weight. Body fat, especially around the belly, is linked to insulin resistance. This explains why many people with prediabetes are also overweight.

Healthy eating

You can't control all risk factors for prediabetes, but some can be mitigated. Lifestyle changes can help you maintain balanced blood sugar levels as well as a healthy weight.

Watch carbs with the glycemic index

The glycemic index (GI) is a tool you can use to determine how a particular food could affect your blood sugar.

Foods that are high on the GI will raise your blood sugar faster. Foods ranked lower on the scale have less effect on your blood sugar spike. Foods with high fiber are low on the GI. Foods that are processed, refined, and void of fiber and nutrients register high on the GI.

Refined carbohydrates rank high on the GI. These are grain products that digest quickly in your stomach. Examples are white bread, russet potatoes, and white rice,

along with soda and juice. Limit these foods whenever possible if you have prediabetes.

Foods that rank medium on the GI are fine to eat. Examples include whole wheat bread and brown rice. Still, they aren't as good as foods that rank low on the GI.

Foods that are low on the GI are best for your blood sugar. Incorporate the following items in your diet:

- ✓ steel-cut oats (not instant oatmeal)
- ✓ stone-ground whole wheat bread
- ✓ nonstarchy vegetables, such as carrots and field greens
- ✓ beans
- ✓ sweet potatoes
- ✓ corn
- ✓ pasta (preferably whole wheat)

Food and nutrition labels don't reveal the GI of a given item. Instead make note of the fiber content listed on the label to help determine a food's GI ranking. Remember to limit saturated fat intake to reduce the risk of developing high cholesterol and heart disease, along with prediabetes.

Eating mixed meals is a great way to lower a food's given GI. For example, if you plan to eat white rice, add vegetables and chicken to slow down the digestion of the grain and minimize spikes.

Portion Control

Good portion control can keep your diet on the low GI. This means you limit the amount of food you eat. Often, portions in the United States are much larger than intended serving sizes. A bagel serving size is usually about one-half, yet many people eat the whole bagel.

Food labels can help you determine how much you're eating. The label will list calories, fat, carbohydrates, and other nutrition information for a particular serving.

If you eat more than the serving listed, it's important to understand how that will affect the nutritional value. A food may have 20 grams of carbohydrate and 150 calories per serving. But if you have two servings, you've consumed 40 grams of carbohydrate and 300 calories.

Eliminating carbohydrates altogether is not necessary. Recent research has shown that a lower-carb diet (less than 40 percent carbs) is associated with the same mortality risk increase as a high-carbohydrate diet (greater than 70 percent carbs).

The study noted minimal risk observed when consuming 50–55 percent carbohydrates in a day. On a 1600-calorie diet, this would equal 200 grams of carbohydrates daily. Spreading intake out evenly throughout the day is best.

This is in line with the National Institute of Health and The Mayo Clinic's recommendation of 45–65 percent of calories coming from carbohydrates daily. Individual carbohydrate needs will vary based on a person's stature and activity level.

Speaking to a dietitian about specific needs is recommended.

One of the best methods to manage portions is to practice mindful eating. Eat when you are hungry. Stop when you are full. Sit, and eat slowly. Focus on the food and flavors.

Eating More Fiber-Rich Foods

Fiber offers several benefits. It helps you feel fuller, longer. Fiber adds bulk to your diet, making bowel movements easier to pass.

Eating fiber-rich foods can make you less likely to overeat. They also help you avoid the "crash" that can come from eating a high-sugar food. These types of foods will often give you a big boost of energy, but make you feel tired shortly after.

Examples of high-fiber foods include:

- ✓ beans and legumes
- ✓ fruits and vegetables that have an edible skin
- ✓ whole-grain breads
- ✓ whole grains such as quinoa or barley
- ✓ whole grain cereals
- ✓ whole wheat pasta
- ✓ Cut out sugary drinks

A single, 12-ounce can of soda can contain 45 grams of carbohydrates. That number is the recommended carbohydrate serving for a meal for women with diabetes. Sugary sodas only offer empty calories that translate to quick-digesting carbohydrates. Water is a better choice to quench your thirst.

Drink Alcohol In Moderation

Moderation is a healthy rule to live by in most instances. Drinking alcohol is no exception. Many alcoholic beverages are dehydrating. Some cocktails may contain high sugar levels that can spike your blood sugar.

According to the American Diabetes Association, women should only have one drink per day while men should limit themselves to no more two drinks per day. Drink servings relate back to portion control. The following are the measurements for an average single drink:

- ✓ 1 bottle of beer (12 fluid ounces)
- ✓ 1 glass of wine (5 fluid ounces)
- ✓ 1 shot of distilled spirits, such as gin, vodka, or whiskey (1.5 fluid ounces)

Keep your drink as simple as possible. Avoid adding sugary juices or liqueurs. Keep a glass of water nearby that you can sip on to prevent dehydration.

Eat Lean Meats

Meat doesn't contain carbohydrates, but it can be a significant source of saturated fat in your diet. Eating a lot of fatty meat can lead to high cholesterol levels.

If you have prediabetes, a diet low in saturated fat and trans fat can help reduce your risk of heart disease. It's recommended that you avoid cuts of meat with visible fat or skin.

Choose protein sources such as the following:

- ✓ chicken without skin
- ✓ egg substitute or egg whites
- ✓ beans and legumes
- ✓ soybean products such as tofu and tempeh
- ✓ fish, such as cod, flounder, haddock, halibut, tuna, or trout
- ✓ lean beef cuts, such as flank steak, ground round, tenderloin, and roast with fat trimmed
- ✓ shellfish, such as crab, lobster, shrimp, or scallops
- ✓ turkey without skin
- ✓ low-fat Greek yogurt

Very lean cuts of meat have about 0 to 1 gram of fat and 35 calories per ounce. High-fat meat choices, such as spareribs, can have more than 7 grams of fat and 100 calories per ounce.

Drinking plenty of water

Water is an important part of any healthy diet. Drink enough water each day to keep you from becoming dehydrated. If you have prediabetes, water is a healthier alternative than sugary sodas, juices, and energy drinks.

The amount of water you should drink every day depends on your body size, activity level, and the climate you live in. You can determine if you're drinking enough water by monitoring the volume of urine when you go. Also make note of the color. Your urine should be pale yellow.

Exercise and diet go together

Exercise is a part of any healthy lifestyle. It's especially important for those with prediabetes.

A lack of physical activity has been linked to increased insulin resistance, according to the National Institute of Diabetes and Digestive and Kidney Diseases (NIDDK). Exercise causes muscles to use glucose for energy, and makes the cells work more effectively with insulin.

The NIDDK recommends exercising five days a week for at least 30 minutes. Exercise doesn't have to be strenuous or overly complicated. Walking, dancing, riding a bicycle, taking an exercise class, or finding another activity you enjoy are all examples of physical activity.

HOW TO BEAT PREDIABETES WITHOUT MAKING YOUR DOCTOR, PHARMACIST OR HEALTH FOOD PRACTITIONER RICH

Wouldn't it be great if you could rejoin the ranks of the healthy without spending a ton of money? I managed to do it. It isn't as hard as you might think.

First of all, the cure for prediabetes can be very inexpensive. In a FAQ on their web site, the American Diabetes Association states:

"Q: What is the treatment for prediabetes? A: Treatment consists of losing a modest amount of weight (5-10 percent of total body weight) through diet and moderate exercise, such as walking, 30 minutes a day, 5 days a week. Don't worry if you can't get to your ideal body weight. A loss of just 10 to 15 pounds can make a huge difference.

It can by very simple and inexpensive to follow this advice, but it is right here that we need a reality check. Sadly, most of us would rather eat what we want, be as lazy as we can get away with being, and then hope to take some magic pill to avoid the consequences. The problem is magic can be very expensive. And more often than not, dietary magic proves to be just an illusion.

It doesn't have to be that way. If done the right way, getting healthy can actually save money. Eating less, decreasing portion sizes and eating high protein foods that satisfy longer, can actually lower your grocery bills. Even if the food budget goes up a bit, it is still cheaper than medicine. Frankly, I would rather financially reward a farmer for proving me good food, than help fund an industry that profits from my sickness.

A healthy diet can save you money, but what about exercise? Gym memberships, special equipment, shoes, clothes, classes, etc., can add up to quite a bit. But, just like a smart diet, exercise can be a bargain. Walking doesn't have to cost anything if you do it right. Instead of buying pills to cure your ills, why not just walk for 30 minutes? It can be as simple as walking out the front door, choosing a direction and noting when you have walked 15 min. Then turn around and come home.

If you want to spend some money to motivate yourself, fine. Some people find joining a gym and working out with a buddy to be just the thing. But driving to a gym, taking the shower there, etc, can eat up a lot of time. When time is short and demands are high, skipping that drive and saving that hour or two becomes very tempting. In choosing an exercise method, a very important question is: "Will I do this every day or regularly without fail?" If the gym, or other more expensive method works for you,

great! You are on your way to better health. Eventually there will be a positive R.O.I (return on investment).

Personally, I like it simple, cheap and inside. Keeping it local or in the house saves a lot of time. This inside method works for me because I can listen to my favorite podcasts, stay dry, and avoid dogs, rain, cars and the mocking stares of kids at the bus-stop. I find that I am more likely to do it every day if it convenient and not subject to interruptions of traffic and tropical storms.

My program has two parts. The first part is weight lifting. I purchased an exercise bench from Sears for about $80 and installed it in my home office. I workout every day (except Sunday), focusing on the different parts of my body, on alternating days, I started light with a lot of reps and added more weights a little at a time. I am up to 85 lb. bench presses, 3 sets of 10 repetitions. For aerobics, I am going cheaper. We have a step inside the house that I have started using. An hour or so after dinner, I usually do 500 steps in 20 min., about the time it takes to watch one of my favorite old shows on Hulu.com. The step is free, the entertainment is free and I lower my blood sugar levels, saving money on medications. That is a "win-win-win" situation. How many "wins" in a row do you need? I can string together a few more, but I think you have enough reasons to stop hiding behind the excuse that weight loss and exercise are difficult and expensive.

OK, so I spent some money on a weight bench. I am not a bit sorry. I might even ask for a $99 "Wii Fit Plus" for Christmas. I might have spent some money, but I am already enjoying benefits of my improved health in my journey towards fitness and haven't spent over $100 in total so far.

The twin pleasures of saving money and getting results are great motivators. Ina addition, my wife Tina and I have started watching "The Biggest Loser" and consequently, are getting tougher on ourselves. Today we walked 35 min. in the park together and planned another walk for later today. But the biggest motivation is seeing that scale go down! I started at 175 about two months ago and weighed in at 152 this morning. That is 23 lbs of success!

The point is, you can get healthy without helping your doctors, pharmacists or health food practitioners get any richer. If you are a cheapskate (I prefer "thrifty") like me, saving some significant cash every month could be just the extra motivation you need to eat right and to lace up those walking shoes and start stepping your way into the land of better health and lower expenses.

PREDIABETES - WHAT WILL YOU DO TO PREVENT TYPE 2 DIABETES?

Prediabetes, or borderline diabetes, is also called impaired glucose tolerance (IGT). When doctors first diagnose anyone with prediabetes, they often treat them the same way as they treat people who have had a heart attack.

Why is this? It might be because you, or your health care provider, did not recognize the signs and symptoms of prediabetes. By the time your blood sugar levels are in the IGT range, the odds are you have had elevated blood sugars for some time. These high levels of sugar in your bloodstream cause damage to your heart and blood vessels.

Prediabetics do not meet the criteria for diabetes type 2, but their blood sugar level is above normal higher than 100mg/dL (5.5mmol/L) as insulin is no longer able to hook up with the sugar and transport it into your cells.

Diagnosis is made by: A fasting plasma glucose reading of greater than 100 to 125mg/dL (5.5 to 6.9mmol/L) taken after eating nothing and drinking only water for eight hours prior to the test, is the current standard for diagnosing prediabetes.

Your doctor might ask you to take a glucose tolerance test (OGTT) which normally takes around two hours. In this test you will have blood drawn before drinking a glucose solution, and then additional measurements are taken hourly. If after two hours the measurement reads 140 to

199mg/dL (7.7 to 11mmol/L)... this points to glucose intolerance and prediabetes.

Another test which is often used is the HbA1c... this test looks at how blood sugar has actually damaged proteins in your blood and gives an overview of your average glucose level over the previous few months. The result is given as a percentage and you would be described as being prediabetic with a reading of 5.7 to 6.9%.

Watch out for a SOS from your body: Yes, blood tests confirm a diagnosis but watch out for these subtle signs and get in early before this condition progresses:

- ✓ stubborn excess weight that stays, no matter what you do
- ✓ urgent cravings for sugary foods including candy, and chips... and many other foods you know are not healthy
- ✓ mood swings that ruin your day and are only relieved by eating

A study reported from Australia, 2007 showed a higher rate of death, and death due to heart disease, in those with prediabetes than in those with normal blood sugar levels. Over ten thousand adults took part in the five year study:

- ✓ almost 1300 had impaired glucose tolerance
- ✓ 610 had impaired fasting glucose
- ✓ 858 had type 2 diabetes at the start of the study

During the study, diabetics were 2.3 times more likely to die from any cause than were healthy people. Subjects with impaired glucose tolerance were 50% more likely to die, and those with impaired fasting glucose were 60% more likely to die than healthy volunteers.

Diabetics and people with impaired fasting glucose were approximately 2.5 times more likely to die of heart disease than those with normal blood sugar levels.

Anyone over 45, particularly if overweight or obese, should be screened for diabetes type 2. This is particularly important if you have:

- ✓ a parent or sibling with diabetes type 2
- ✓ high cholesterol or high blood pressure
- ✓ a history of gestational diabetes or gave birth to a baby weighing over 9 pounds
- ✓ a sedentary lifestyle
- ✓ a diet low in fiber, high in processed foods and simple carbohydrates

As bad as this all sounds, there is much you can do to change the course of your health. This is a wake-up call... diabetes type 2 is a serious condition no action will lead to full blown type 2 diabetes.

Would you like more information about alternative ways to handle your type 2 diabetes?

PREDIABETES: 7 STEPS TO TAKE NOW

What to do to stop prediabetes from becoming diabetes.

Getting diagnosed with prediabetes is a serious wake-up call, but it doesn't have to mean you will definitely get diabetes. There is still time to turn things around.

"It's an opportunity to initiate lifestyle changes or treatments, and potentially retard progression to diabetes or even prevent diabetes," says Gregg Gerety, MD, chief of endocrinology at St. Peter's Hospital in Albany, N.Y.

Making these seven changes in your daily habits is a good way to start.

Move More

Becoming more active is one of the best things you can do to make diabetes less likely. If it's been a while since you exercised, start by building more activity into your routine by taking the stairs or doing some stretching during TV commercials, says Patti Geil, MS, RD, author of

"Physical activity is an essential part of the treatment plan for prediabetes, because it lowers blood glucose levels and decreases body fat," Geil says.

Live Better With MS - Is there room for improvement?

Take this WebMD assessment and get personalized tips to help live your life with MS to the fullest.

Healthy Living With Hepatitis C

Ideally, you should exercise at least 30 minutes a day, five days a week. Let your doctor know about your exercise plans and ask if you have any limitations.

Lower Your Weight

If you're overweight, you might not have to lose as much as you think to make a difference.

In one study, people who had prediabetes and lost 5% to 7% of their body weight (just 10-14 pounds in someone who weights 200 pounds) cut their chances of getting diabetes by 58%.

See Your Doctor More Often

See your doctor every three to six months, Gerety says.

If you're doing well, you can get positive reinforcement from your doctor. If it's not going so well, your doctor can help you get back on track.

"Patients like some tangible evidence of success or failure," Gerety says.

Eat Better

Load up on vegetables, especially the less-starchy kinds such as spinach and other leafy greens, broccoli, carrots, and green beans. Aim for at least three servings a day.

Add more high-fiber foods into your day.

Enjoy fruits in moderation - 1 to 3 servings per day.

Choose whole-grain foods instead of processed grains for example, brown rice instead of white rice.

Also, swap out high-calorie foods. "Drink skim milk rather than whole milk, diet soda rather than regular soda," Geil says. "Choose lower-fat versions of cheese, yogurt, and salad dressings."

Instead of snacking on high-fat, high-calorie chips and desserts, choose fresh fruit, or whole wheat crackers with peanut butter or low-fat cheese, Geil says.

Make Sleep A Priority

Not getting enough sleep regularly makes losing weight harder, says Theresa Garnero, author of Your First Year With Diabetes.

A sleep shortfall also makes it harder for your body to use insulin effectively and may make type 2 diabetes more likely.

Set good sleep habits. Go to bed and wake up at the same time every day. Relax before you turn out the lights. Don't watch TV or use your computer or smartphone when you're trying to fall asleep. Avoid caffeine after lunch if you have trouble sleeping.

Get Support.

Losing weight, eating a healthy diet, and exercising regularly is easier if you have people helping you out, holding you accountable, and cheering you on, says Ronald T. Ackermann, MD, MPH, an associate professor of medicine at Indiana University School of Medicine.

Consider joining a group where you can pursue a healthier lifestyle in the company of others with similar goals.

A certified diabetes educator may also help you learn about what you need to do to prevent your prediabetes from becoming diabetes. You can find one through the American Association of Diabetes Educators.

Choose And Commit

Having the right mind-set can help.

Accept that you won't do things perfectly every day, but pledge to do your best most of the time.

"Make a conscious choice to be consistent with everyday activities that are in the best interest of your health," Garnero says. "Tell yourself, 'I'm going to give it my best. I'm going to make small changes over time.'

MEAL PLANS FOR DIABETES AND PRE-DIABETES

A healthy eating plan for Type 2 Diabetes is the same recommendation for most of us. There is no need to buy 'special foods' or cook separate meals. Your daily food intake should include the following foods:

- ✓ 5-6 serves of breads and cereals and other starchy foods.
- ✓ 2-3 serves fruit.
- ✓ 5 or more serves of vegetables.
- ✓ 2-3 serves of milk products or alternatives.
- ✓ 1-2 serves meat or vegetarian alternatives.
- ✓ 2-3 serves of fats and oils

This daily food guide is based on a 60 years plus overweight active individual.

How much is in a serve?

The following food groups provide a guide to a serving size of foods that are nutritionally similar (e.g. 1 slice of bread has similar carbohydrate amount to ⅓ cup of cooked rice). Foods can be swapped or exchanged for another within the same group.

Breads, cereals and other starchy foods:

- ✓ 1 slice of whole grain bread (30 – 35 g)
- ✓ ⅓ cup natural muesli (30 – 35g)
- ✓ ¼ cup rolled oats (30 g)
- ✓ 2 breakfast wheat biscuits (30 g)

- ✓ ⅓ cup cooked rice (65g)
- ✓ ½ cup cooked pasta or noodles (75g)
- ✓ ⅓ cup pearl barley (65g)
- ✓ ½ cup cooked kidney beans, chickpeas, kidney beans, borlotti beans etc (85g)
- ✓ ¾ cup cooked lentils (145g)
- ✓ 1 medium potato or 2 new/baby potatoes (such as Carisma™) (125g)
- ✓ ¾ cup diced sweet potato (110g)
- ✓ ½ large ear of corn or ½ cup corn kernels (90g)

Fruit:

- ✓ 1 medium piece of fruit (apple, orange, banana)
- ✓ 2 small pieces of fruit (apricot, plum, kiwi fruit)
- ✓ ½ cup canned fruit (120g)
- ✓ 20 g dried fruit (6 apricot halves, 6 prunes or dates, 1 ½ Tbs sultanas)
- ✓ ½ cup juice (150ml)

Vegetables:

- ✓ ½ cup cooked vegetables
- ✓ 1 cup raw leafy salad greens
- ✓ 1 cup of vegetable soup
- ✓ Milk and dairy alternatives:
- ✓ 1 cup of reduced fat milk (125ml)
- ✓ 200g tub of reduced fat yoghurt
- ✓ 1 cup of buttermilk (250ml)
- ✓ 1 cup of calcium fortified soy drink
- ✓ 40g reduced fat hard cheese

Meat and alternatives:

- ✓ 100g (raw weight) of lean meat or chicken

- ✓ 150g raw fish
- ✓ 100g drained canned fish
- ✓ 200g tofu
- ✓ 1 cup cooked beans such as soybeans
- ✓ 60g reduced fat cheese
- ✓ 2 eggs

Fats And Oils:

- ✓ 2 tsp mono or poly unsaturated oil
- ✓ 2 tsp mono or polyunsaturated margarine
- ✓ ¼ (50g) avocado
- ✓ 20 g nuts
- ✓ 3 tsp peanut spread
- ✓ 1 Tbs oil based salad dressing

Some hints and tips to include high protein, low GI foods at each meal.

Breakfast

Kick start your day with a good breakfast to help sustain your energy levels and concentration throughout the morning. A healthy breakfast will prime your metabolism to start burning fat right away. A higher protein lower GI breakfast is an ideal food combo to get you off to a healthy start:

Smart Carbs – traditional oats, natural muesli, low GI breakfast cereals, toast made with grainy low GI breads or authentic sourdough, fruit loaf; baked beans or canned sweetcorn.

Protein Power – reduced fat milk or yoghurt on their own or made into a fruit smoothie, eggs, ricotta or cottage cheese, tofu, nuts and nut spread, lean slices of ham or bacon and smoked salmon.

Fruit and Vegetables – fresh, frozen or canned fruit and vegetables, dried fruit, small amount of fresh fruit and vegetable juice, grilled tomatoes, or cooked spinach and mushrooms.

- ✓ Go Low with simple swaps
- ✓ Instead of Enjoy
- ✓ Flaked and puffed breakfast cereals
- ✓ Natural muesli
- ✓ Instant Oats/Porridge
- ✓ Porridge or Bircher muesli made with traditional oats or steel cut oats
- ✓ Muffin or Banana Bread
- ✓ Toasted fruit breads
- ✓ White or wholemeal toast
- ✓ Dense grainy or authentic sourdough toast

Lunch

You'll have a more productive afternoon without cravings or feeling drowsy if you make time for lunch. Choose foods from each group. A serving of beans, lentils and yoghurt will also provide both carbs and protein for longer lasting energy.

Smart carbs – dense grain and seeded or authentic sourdough breads and rolls, bean salad or baked beans, lentil soups, 'al dente' pasta (with vegetable or tomato based sauce), noodles (not fried), low GI rice such as SunRice® Doongara™ or Basmati, corn on the cob, tub of yoghurt.

Protein Power – sandwich fillings such as canned salmon or

tuna, lean ham or rare roast beef, egg/frittata slice, chargrilled chicken or beef skewers.

Fruit and Vegetables – add salad to sandwiches, rolls or wraps, tubs of garden, Greek or Asian salad, vegetable soup (not laksa), stir fry vegetables, fresh rice paper rolls, tubs of fruit salad, fruit smoothie or vegetable juice.

Go Low with some simple swaps

Instead of Enjoy

- ✓ White bread, rolls or hamburger buns
- ✓ Dense grain and seeded or authentic sourdough breads and rolls
- ✓ Filled bagels or baguettes
- ✓ Mission white corn tortilla wraps with kebabs, tabbouli and hummus
- ✓ Hot chips
- ✓ Hot corn on the cob; baked Carisma™ potato
- ✓ Pizza
- ✓ Sourdough bruschetta
- ✓ Fried rice
- ✓ Long or short soup with noodles or wontons

Dinner

Taking time for dinner is an integral part of healthy eating. Turn off the TV people who watch TV while eating tend to mindlessly eat more. If you are rushed after work with no time to cook, stock you fridge and cupboards on the weekend to whip up a meal. Choose foods from each of the food groups. Beans, split peas and lentils provide both carbs and protein.

Smart carbs – (¼ dinner plate) – lower GI potatoes such as Carisma or orange fleshed sweet potato, parsnips, butternut pumpkin; pasta or noodles; low GI rice such as SunRice® Doongara™ or lower GI Basmati; quinoa, pearl barley, corn on the cob, beans, split peas and lentils.

Protein Power – (¼ dinner plate) – fish or seafood, fresh or canned, lean meat or poultry, eggs or tofu.

Fruit and Vegetables – (½ dinner plate) – plenty of salads and vegetables (it's your best chance to get in your 5 serves of veggies). Still hungry? Round off with a piece of fruit.

PREDIABETES, DIABETES TYPE 1 AND DIABETES TYPE 2 ALL FEATURE PROGRESSIVE GLYCATION OF MOLECULES

Glycation. Glycation is a random reaction between the ordinary glucose molecule and any tissue or any macromolecule in our bodies. Glycation is not enzyme-directed. It is not enzyme-facilitated. Glycation serves no positive purpose. Glycation is a chemical reaction between a substance - glucose - which has the property of sharing an electron with another molecule - and a receiving molecule, most usually a protein or lipoprotein. A glycation event is an irreversible union of glucose with a receptive molecule. Receptive molecules include hemoglobin, capillary endothelial cell membrane proteins, and structural membrane proteins of numerous organs, such as kidneys and nerves. Glycation reactions in our bodies occur when glucose molecules circulate too long in the blood stream - having not been transported into cells and tissues by insulin. How long is too long? Too long most certainly is greater than 3 hours. Even two hours can be too long. This random attachment of glucose changes the basic nature of the proteins and membranes. Glycation is undesirable, for it initiates and perpetuates disease on the organs affected.

Type 1 Diabetes Mellitus. Type 1 Diabetes Mellitus features relative insulin lack or insulin deficiency as its basic root cause. Insulin is present but in sub-normal concentrations. Insulin secretion in response to a glucose-containing meal is low, sluggish, and sub-normal, as well. The basic problem resides at the pancreas beta-cell, which are the cells where insulin is manufactured and secreted in response to glucose surges in our blood stream. Physicians can and do prescribe various insulin forms and dosages to repair and remedy the insulin deficiencies. But, a basic second problem can persist - glucose is not transported into target organ cells as promptly as would occur in the perfectly healthy state.

Hence, blood glucose concentrations can be lowered with prescribed insulin preparations, but glucose absorbed from our meals still circulates too long and at higher than normal concentrations. Then, glycation events result. Tissue membranes are affected. Capillary wall membranes are affected. Organ disease results and progresses.

Type 2 Diabetes Mellitus. Type 2 Diabetes Mellitus features resistance to insulin action at the target tissue level. Insulin production and insulin secretion by the pancreas beta-cells is not below normal. In fact, insulin secretion is either normal or above normal. Most commonly, insulin secretion and presence rises in a biologic attempt to overcome the insulin resistance and to transport circulating glucose into the target tissues. Physicians will prescribe various pill forms of diabetes medications that aim to improve blood glucose and will even add various forms of insulin on top

of the already present natural insulin. These interventions can help. Still, though, the blood stream glucose concentrations will linger in higher-than-normal ranges, perpetrating and perpetuating glycation events at various sites.

Prediabetes. Prediabetes is a recognizable condition where an individual experiences elevated blood glucose concentrations after a long fasting period, or will exhibit higher-than-physiologically normal glycated hemoglobin levels. Yes, elevated glycated hemoglobin events labels a person as being prediabetic. The elevated glycated hemoglobin concentration is not severe, but it is real. Hence, the person is diagnosed with prediabetes. Why call this prediabetes if glycation events are super-normal? What not call this condition Type 3 Diabetes? Well, prediabetes is a condition that does not mandate a diabetic pill or an insulin prescription. Prediabetes can be reversed and normalized with diet pattern alterations, with sustained weight loss, and with regular exercise. Nevertheless, prediabetes features glycation events, which are known to be harmful if left to progress and accumulate.

Actions. All three of these metabolic disorders are real. All three feature abnormalities of glucose metabolism. All three feature glycation events. The glycation events are the harmful and hurtful consequences of altered glucose metabolism. Action is essential. Action begins with awareness and with understanding. Action hinges on consuming small and smaller quantities of simple carbohydrates at any and every meal, of avoiding sugary snacks and drinks, and obtaining expert diagnosis, counsel and management of your particular condition. Know this and do this.

What Should You Eat If You Have Diabetes?

In truth, a diet aimed at reducing the risks of diabetes is really nothing more than a nutritionally-balanced meal plan aimed at supporting maintaining blood sugar levels within range and supporting a healthy weight.

For those with prediabetes or type 2 diabetes, the main focus of a diabetes-focused diet is being attentive to your weight.2 That said, a diabetic diet is simply an eating approach that works to keep you healthy, and so is not reserved only for people with diabetes. Your whole family can enjoy the same meals and snacks, regardless of whether others have diabetes or not.

Yes There are a few food decisions that will matter more if you do have diabetes. We provide you with some general guidelines to help you understand how much and how often to eat in order to maintain steady blood sugar levels. And, these recommendations hold true for anyone who has diabetes: type 1 diabetes and type 2 diabetes, as well as prediabetes and gestational diabetes.1

Diet really does matter, a lot!

In fact, if you were recently diagnosed with prediabetes or type 2 diabetes, by decreasing your weight by about 10%, you may even reverse your diabetes, putting it into remission.3,4

ADOPTING A DIABETES DIET PLAN FOR LONG-TERM HEALTH

By becoming a bit more savvy about the effect that foods, especially carbs, can have on your blood sugar, you will want to know how and why to adjust your food choices; you can feel so much better in the process.

It may ease your mind to know you will be able to incorporate your favorite foods into a healthy diet while being mindful of your diabetes diet goals (eg, healthy weight, steady blood glucose levels, good blood pressure). For many people, at least initially, this may seem harder than it should be and that's understandable; after all, it can seem very, very challenging to change current eating habits and find the right food rhythm to fit your lifestyle.

You don't have to go it alone Seek advice from a registered dietitian (RD) or certified diabetes educator (CDE) who has the right training to help you come up with an individualized meal plan that will help you meet your self-management goals, get the nutrition you need, and show you how you can incorporate some of your favorite foods into your diet so that you continue to enjoy eating. Hopefully, your doctor has someone on the team, but if not, call your health insurer to ask for the names of a few in-network RD/CDEs.2

There are also virtual coaching programs that appear very effective; this means you can get individualized dietary guidance at home or at work. Most health insurance companies will cover the cost of diabetic diet counseling so ask your doctor for a prescription so cost doesn't hold you back.

"While the idea of changing your diet can be confusing and overwhelming at first, research shows that making healthy lifestyle choices can help you manage your blood sugar levels in the short term and may even prevent many of the long-term health complications associated with diabetes," says Lori Zanini, RD, CDE, and author of The Diabetes Cookbook and Meal Plan for the Newly Diagnosed.

Although you can include most foods in a diabetic diet, you do need to pay most attention to particularly to the types of carbohydrates you choose in order to prevent spikes, or unhealthy increases, in your blood sugar.

Foods high in simple carbohydrates mostly from added sugars (ie, cane sugar, brown sugar, maple syrup, honey) and refined grains (especially white flour and white rice) as foods containing these ingredients will cause your blood sugar levels to rise more quickly than foods that contain fiber, such as 100% whole wheat and oats.

"Everyone is different and, ultimately, you know best how your body responds to different types of foods, so you may have to make individual adjustments when cooking at home, eating out, or attending celebrations," Ms. Zanini points out. "You may find that some processed, high-carb foods, like commercial breakfast cereals and plain white rice, are just too "spiky" for you and it's best to stay away from them and find reasonable substitutes."

MANAGING HIGH CHOLESTEROL WHEN YOU HAVE DIABETES

Type 2 diabetes often goes hand-in-hand with unhealthy cholesterol levels. Even someone with diabetes who has good control of their blood glucose is more likely than otherwise healthy people to develop any or all of several cholesterol problems that increase the risk of atherosclerosis and other cardiovascular problems, according to the Cleveland Clinic.

If you have diabetes, you've already made changes to your diet and lifestyle that are targeted to keeping your blood glucose (blood sugar) levels steady. But given the increased risk of heart problems associated with diabetes, you may want to also take steps to keep your cholesterol levels steady as well.

Aspects of Cholesterol Problems

In and of itself, cholesterol is not a bad thing: It's present in every cell in the body and does a lot of good supporting the production of hormones, digestion, and converting sunlight into vitamin D. Approximately 75 percent of the cholesterol present in the blood is produced by the liver, but the rest is derived from the diet, which is why making dietary changes is an effective way to keep cholesterol levels healthy.

There are two types of cholesterol:

Low-density lipoprotein (LDL) cholesterol is regarded as

"bad cholesterol." It's the soft, waxy stuff that can accumulate in the bloodstream and interfere with the flow of blood.

High-density lipoprotein (HDL) the so-called "good cholesterol"helps keep blood vessels clear by carrying LDL cholesterol to the liver for disposal.

In addition to cholesterol, the levels of triglycerides (fats) in the body are important to heart health and so usually are considered a key aspect of a person's overall blood cholesterol "profile."

Cholesterol Level Guidelines for Adults 20 and Older

Healthy Eating Guidelines

Managing both diabetes and cholesterol levels is a matter of being careful about the amounts of carbohydrates, cholesterol, and saturated fats in your diet, as well as making sure you're getting enough of certain nutrients that can help to improve your blood sugar and cholesterol levels.

Total Carbohydrates

There are several types of carbs: Of particular importance are complex carbs (a.k.a. starches), found in foods like legumes, whole grains, starchy vegetables, pasta, and bread, and simple carbs. Simple carbs are, simply, sugars.

For most people with diabetes, especially those who take insulin and are monitoring their blood sugar levels before and after meals, there's no hard-and-fast number of ideal carbs per day: That will depend on the results of each meter reading.

However, according to the National Institute of Diabetes and Digestive and Kidney Diseases (NIDDK), the recommended carbohydrate intake for most people is between 45 percent and 65 percent of total calories from carbohydrates, with the exception of those who are physically inactivie or on low-calorie diets.

For someone following an 1,800-calorie diet, that would mean getting 202.5 grams of carbs each day, based on the fact that there are four calories per one gram of carbohydrate.

Added Sugar

Sugar crops up in the diet in two ways: It's a natural component of fresh fruit, for example. But it also shows up as an additive, often surreptitiously, in items like fruit drinks and even condiments such as ketchup and barbecue sauce. The 2015-2020 Dietary Guidelines for Americans, developed by the Department of Health and Human Services and the U.S. Food and Drug Administration (USDA), recommends keeping added sugar to fewer than 10 percent of calories each day.

Saturated Fat

Saturated fats, found in foods such as animal protein and processed meats, certain plant oils, dairy products, and pre-packages snacks, are known to raise the levels of LDL cholesterol in the body. The Dietary Guidelines for America advise getting fewer than 10 percent of total daily calories from saturated fat, while the American Heart Association (AHA), recommends that less than 5 percent to 6 percent of daily calories consist of saturated fat. For someone following a 2,000-calorie diet, that would come to no more than 120 calories worth of saturated fat, or around 13 grams.

Trans Fat

This is an especially bad type of saturated fat that results from the heating of liquid vegetable oils (hydrogenation), a process done to unnaturally give foods a longer shelf life. It's used in margarine, processed snack foods and baked goods, and for frying. The AHA recommends limiting trans fat to less than 2 grams per day.

In addition to following the dietary guidelines set out for general health and also monitoring your glucose to determine how certain foods, especially carbs, affect your blood levels, there are other effective ways to manage diabetes and maintain healthy cholesterol levels.

Eat More Fiber

Fiber is the part of plants that can't be digested. Although it's very filling, it won't add calories because the body can't absorb it, making it useful for weight loss. What's more, soluble fiber, found in foods like beans, apples, and oatmeal, helps lower LDL cholesterol and keep blood glucose levels steady.

A good rule of thumb for getting ample fiber at each meal is to fill half your plate with non-starchy vegetables—anything from artichokes and asparagus to turnips and zucchini. These are rich in fiber (as well as phytonutrients that can further help protect your overall health).

Aim to increase the amount of fiber you eat every day

gradually, to at least 25 grams per day if you're a woman and 38 grams per day if you're a man.

Choose Good Fats Over Bad Fats

Fat is an important nutrient, necessary for energy and hormone production, vitamin absorption, maintaining the membrane integrity of every cell in our body, and growth and development. According to the Dietary Reference Intakes published by the USDA, 20 percent to 35 percent of calories should come from fat. But when it comes to dietary fat, not all types are created equal.

As noted above, saturated fats contribute to high levels of LDL cholesterol, as do the trans fats in fried foods and baked goods. At the same time, however, monounsaturated fats, which are found in olives, olive oil, and certain nuts and seeds, actually help lower blood cholesterol levels.

Another type of good fat, the polyunsaturated fat in fatty fish like salmon and trough, as well as flaxseeds and walnuts, are rich in omega-3 fatty acids that play a significant role in reducing overall blood cholesterol and triglyceride levels.

Lose Weight

If you're overweight or obese, losing just 10 to 15 pounds can have a tremendously positive effect on both your diabetes and your cholesterol levels by helping to lower your blood glucose, blood pressure, and improve your blood fats. You may even be able to cut down on your medications.

One of the best ways to begin a safe and effective weight loss plan tailored to you is to keep a record of what you eat, how much you eat, and around what time you eat for three days, ideally two weekdays and one weekend. You can then have a registered dietitian analyze it (or use and online program) to determine the average number of calories you are eating and to learn other patterns, such as how many vegetables you're eating (or not eating), and the main kinds of fat in your diet.

Armed with this information, you'll be able to see how many fewer calories you should eat in order to lose weight at a slow and steady rate, and what

foods you should cut back on or steer clear of in order to eat less added sugar and saturated fats.

Get On Your Feet

Physical activity burns calories, which is why exercise is always recommended as part of a weight-loss plan particularly for someone with diabetes.

Exercise also has been found to help lower total cholesterol levels. What kind? In studies, a combination of aerobic exercise and strength-training has been found ideal.

As for how much and how often you should work out, the AHA advises 150 minutes per week of moderate-intensity aerobic activity, or 75 minutes per week of vigorous aerobic activity, or a combination of both, preferably spread throughout the week. You'll gain even more benefits by being active at least 300 minutes (five hours) per week. Add moderate- to high-intensity muscle-strengthening activity at least two days per week.

If that sounds like a lot to start, don't be discouraged: Any physical activity is better than nothing, even if it's just taking the stairs instead of the elevator, or walking around the block. And if you find it hard to exercise for long periods at a time, divide it up into shorter sessions—10 or 15 minutes throughout the day.

Kick The Habit

If you smoke, quitting will impact both your HDL and LDL cholesterol levels for the good. Cigarette smoking is linked to higher cholesterol levels as well as the formation of a damaging form of LDL called oxidized LDL, which contributes to atherosclerosis. In fact, as soon as you stop smoking your cholesterol levels will begin to decrease, research shows. With each month after quitting, LDL levels continue to lower, even partially reversing the effects of smoking on cholesterol after just 90 days

NORMAL BLOOD SUGAR - WHAT IS A NORMAL BLOOD SUGAR?

The normal blood sugar levels of people with diabetes is between 80-90 mg/dL before meals and may rise up to 120 mg/dL or a little more after they eat, depending on what kind of food they had.

Untreated or undertreated diabetes means persistently high blood sugars, which can cause horrible arterial blockages, resulting in strokes and heart attacks. High blood sugars also cause nerve damage, with burning leg pain that eventually gives way to numbness. This, combined with the arterial blockages, can result in deformities and dead tissue, which is why many people with diabetes end up with amputations. The tiny blood vessels to the retina are also affected, which can cause blindness. And don't forget the kidneys, which are especially susceptible to the damage caused by high blood sugar. Diabetes is a leading cause of kidney failure requiring dialysis and/or kidney transplant. But wait! There's more. High blood sugar impairs the white blood cell function critical to a healthy immune system, and sugar is a great source of energy for invading bacteria and fungi. These factors put folks at risk of nasty infections of all kinds.

These facts scare me. Not just because I'm the doctor who gets to help manage these not-fun issues, but because I'm of Latina descent and diabetes runs in my own family. I'm at risk too.

So, what can we do? If we know who is at risk for diabetes, and it takes years to develop, we should be able to prevent it, right? Right!

RegardLess of what you've eaten, a blood sugar level above 140 mg/dL is NOT normal and needs to be checked out. Any suspicion of high blood sugar level should be verified by testing your fasting blood sugar level. It's better to know for sure if you have diabetes or prediabetes, so you can take some action. Even if the test shows only a slightly increased risk for diabetes, you should start working on maintaining a healthy weight, eating a healthy diet and exercising regularly.

Someone who does not have diabetes never has a blood sugar above 140 mg/dL - never, not even after eating the entire jar of Ben and Jerry ice cream with syrup. Not even after drinking ten cups of soda.

When you are diagnosed with diabetes or even prediabetes, you need to quickly get familiar with glucose test numbers because you may be checking your own sugar levels several times per day. Interpreting these numbers quickly becomes automatic.

- ✓ Less than 100 mg/dL: Fasting (before breakfast) blood glucose level - Normal level. Optimal blood sugar level is between 80-90 mg/dL
- ✓ 100 mg/dL to 125 mg/dL: Fasting (before breakfast) blood glucose level - Prediabetes
- ✓ Above 125 mg/dL: Fasting (before breakfast) blood glucose level - Diabetes.
- ✓ 140 mg/dL to 200 mg/dL: Random blood glucose level - Possibly diabetes.
- ✓ Above 200 mg/dL: Random blood glucose level with symptoms of thirst, excessive urination, weight loss - Diabetes.

If you have been diagnosed with diabetes or prediabetes, you may be feeling scared or confused, but do not panic. And, even more importantly, do not go into denial. Type 2 diabetes can be controlled and even reversed.

The sooner you get help and start making changes to your diet and life-habits, the better off you will be. Although initially it may feel like your entire life has been taken over by the disease, do not despair. With time healthy living habits will become your second nature.

What you should know is you can prevent, and even reverse diabetes because the disease is influenced by your lifestyle choices, most importantly diet and exercise.

TYPE 2 DIABETES - THE DEVELOPMENT OF TYPE 2 DIABETES FROM PREDIABETES

Impaired fasting glucose, or prediabetes, is a condition in which people do not process sugar normally and their blood sugar levels are higher than normal, but full-blown Type 2 diabetes has not yet been diagnosed. Researchers at the National University of Singapore studied how long it would take for impaired fasting glucose to progress to full-blown Type 2 diabetes. The results of their work were published in the Journal of Diabetes in October 2011.

Four hundred and ninety volunteers with a diagnosis of impaired fasting glucose were included in the study and followed for 1.65 years. At the end of that time:

85 volunteers had progressed to full-blown Type 2 diabetes.

The annual rate of progression from impaired fasting glucose to diabetes was 6.8 per cent. The volunteers found to have the highest blood sugar levels and those with the highest body mass indexes... had the highest rates of progression to diabetes.

Impaired fasting glucose is actually diagnosed when blood sugar after an overnight fast is 100 to 125 mg/dL (5.5 to 6.9 mmol/L). When risk factors such as:

- ✓ obesity,
- ✓ age of 50 or higher,
- ✓ a sedentary lifestyle, or

✓ a family history of Type 2 diabetes

is present, drawing a blood sugar level should be considered. If the blood sugar level indicates prediabetes, then a plan can be undertaken to prevent its progression to full-blown Type 2 diabetes.

Normal body mass index is between 18.5 and 24.9. If it is 25 or higher, it is time to bring it down within normal limits to prevent not only diabetes but heart and blood vessel disease and many other conditions.

A combination of diet and exercise is the best way to normalize a high body weight.

✓ a good diet, high in vitamins, minerals, antioxidants and fiber and low in calories, will not only cause the body to burn fat for energy, but will help curb your appetite and improve your good general health.
✓ food cravings are often caused by unmet needs for nutrients, so supplying what the body needs can help to curb cravings.
✓ vegan and vegetarian diets are good for providing bulk and nutrients without a lot of calories.

Physical activity not only causes the body to burn calories, but increases muscle mass.

✓ muscles burn more calories at rest than fat does, so building up muscles will help to burn calories all day long.
✓ exercise also helps to protect against heart and blood vessel disease and helps keep the body perfused with a good blood supply.

✓ even the skin takes on a healthier appearance when a sedentary lifestyle is shed for a more physically active one, because skin cells are able to get the oxygen and nutrients they need.

WHAT TO DO WHEN ONE HAS PRE-DIABETES SYMPTOMS

Most of the people who develop diabetes also experience pre-diabetes symptoms. If a person is concerned with his or her health, knowing these signs will avoid being diagnosed with diabetes in the long run. Unlike the actual diabetes, the symptoms of pre-diabetes indicate that a person's blood sugar levels are elevated, but not enough to indicate the onset of diabetes. To illustrate this point, a blood sugar level of 100 to 126 milligrams is an indicator that a person has symptoms of pre-diabetes. However, a person has to be alarmed because this could only mean that he or she has developed resistance to insulin making him or her vulnerable to developing diabetes.

A give-away of pre-diabetes symptoms is a diet that is rich in carbohydrates and a person who abuses his or her diet may develop these symptoms quite quickly. This can be tricky though because there are people who eat excess amounts of carbohydrates, but their blood sugar reading is maintained at less than 100 milligrams. However, there are tell-tale signs that people have to reduce their intake of carbohydrates and sugar and these are: heartburn when one is asleep, gas pain, irregular bowel movement, stool issues like constipation and diarrhea. Sleep apnea is usually related to being overweight and this is marked with difficulty in breathing. Too many sweets can make one feel light-headed or dizzy, so he or she should limit his or her intake of chocolates, candy bars, and other foods that are rich in sugar.

An alarming sign would be unchanged eating habits and the person will notice that he or she gained ten pounds all of a sudden without even trying. Moreover, that person has difficulty in getting rid of the excess poundage even if he or she consumes less food or exercises. Also, an individual feels tired even if he or she has enough sleep and fatigue can set in whenever that person exercises. Pre-diabetes symptoms also include persistent pain in the joints, muscles or a feeling of stiffness especially in the morning, which only means that arthritis has set in so people who are obese should be wary of their high fat diet. After all that is said and done, the only way a person

can prevent the onset of pre-diabetes is to lower carbohydrate intake and check out his or her blood sugar with a glucometer. This device will help a person control his or her intake of food.

PREDIABETES AND OBESITY, THE TRUTH ABOUT LOSING WEIGHT

The link between prediabetes and obesity has been proven. Of course, every obese person is not a type 2 diabetic, and it is possible to be diabetic without being overweight.

But obesity increases the risk of developing prediabetes. As obesity becomes a world-wide problem the link cannot be ignored.

Statistically Speaking

In 2000 there were over 1.1 billion overweight individuals in the world, and 312 million were estimated to be obese. The numbers have tripled in areas where the Western diet has recently replaced traditional local foods.

Places like the Middle East, Pacific Islands, India, Southeast Asia and China are seeing this happen. Diabetics are expected to increase from 84 million in 2000 to 228 million in 2030.

The connection between obesity and our Western diet seems clear. When fast food chains flooded Australia, type 2 diabetes cases shot up there, and four times faster among the aborigines as the rest of the country.

Why Is Our Western Diet So Bad?

Eating convenience foods, added sugar products and fast food leads to high triglycerides even in people who are not overweight. Heart and blood vessel problems as well as inflammatory syndromes have been linked to high triglycerides.

Your pancreas, especially the beta cells that control how your body handles food, are thrown out of balance by high triglycerides and inflammation. Next you see fat deposits increase, which leads to abdominal obesity and insulin resistance.

In most cases insulin resistance will become prediabetes even without adding genetic factors. The greater the obesity the faster insulin resistance will push you into type 2 diabetes.

When insulin resistant cells send out a message that they need glucose, the liver responds, making matters worse. Beta cells are already under attack from an inflammatory diet. As the sick beta cells try to restore order by making more insulin, they become weaker and weaker.

The progression from prediabetes and obesity to full-blown type 2 diabetes is slow, so there is time to do something about it. But you cannot waste time by doing things that won't work.

Diets Cannot End Obesity

When you think about fighting prediabetes and obesity your first thought is probably to diet. But which one should you pick? Every man-made diet has its success stories. There are so many choices.

Maybe this will help you decide. Studies have been carried

on for many years comparing popular diets. Researchers follow all of them from low-calorie to Atkins to every other modern diet. Here's what they found.

After one year, all of the diets performed equally well. Not one of them was better than another for long-term weight loss. Every dieter succeeded or failed based on one question. Did they stay on the diet or quit?

So weight loss success came from sticking with it. Turn that statement around and you see the truth. It is not dieting that works, but making a permanent change in what you eat and how much. This is what will stop prediabetes and obesity.

Why Dieting Won't Work

I hate the word dieting. It implies that we can "go on a diet" for a while and then return to our normal habits. That is the real reason diets don't work. Following dieters over many years has proved it.

People who study prediabetes and obesity have published their work in medical journals meant for the eyes of doctors. The articles urge doctors to stop asking their obese diabetic patients to expect a normal BMI (fat to muscle ratio.

Everyone knows that a normal BMI has led to type 2 diabetic remission in some pretty famous people who were once obese. So why are they advising doctors not to set this goal for their patients?

It is because these researchers are looking at the average results for diabetics who take doctors' advice and go on a diet. They find that most dieters lose 5-10% of their starting weight in the first six months and then level off. On average they keep about half of the weight loss for another six months and do not continue to lose weight at all.

Why do diabetic dieters quit trying? The problem seems to be with high expectations. Doctors urge you to get to your optimal BMI, so you try a low calorie or low carb diet, or maybe a portion controlled diet from the frozen foods section of the grocery store.

There is no limit to the things you can find to try. But every diet works best in the first few months and then levels off. You hit a plateau, or you gain weight from your diabetic medications.

In the beginning of your diabetic journey, out of control blood sugar causes weight loss no matter how much you eat. But as your blood sugar is forced to return to normal by medications, weight gain is a common side effect.

If you have to take insulin, as I do, it will make you hungrier. Another problem is that insulin tells your body to store calories as fat. That is what it was designed to do.

Losing weight becomes a real struggle. Weight loss espectations that are not realistic lead to giving up. And most people do give up. The average length of most diets is six months to a year.

The best way to fight obesity is to forget about dieting. Don't fall into the trap of losing weight without changing habits. Any weight you lose will not stay off.

Even people who go through the pain of gastric surgery

often gain back every pound they lose. Believe it or not, fighting obesity is not about weight loss. It is about changing the things that made us obese.

When we understand this, the weight we lose will be a great thermometer to gauge how we are changing, not a goal we try to reach so we can go back to our old ways.

The path out of prediabetes and obesity includes eating mostly fresh whole foods, not processed meals and fast food fare. Change takes time, but every permanent change in the way you eat will make you healthier.

FIVE TIPS FOR BEATING DIABETES AND OBESITY

If you are going to beat obesity, is important to set realistic milestones for your weight loss. Losing and maintaining 10% of your starting weight will not give you the diabetic cure of a perfect BMI, but it will add years to your life.

Increase your physical activity. Exercise will increase your quality of life as well as help you continue to lose weight and keep it off for years. Adding exercise does end prediabetes and obesity if you don't stop doing it.

Don't give up when your weight won't budge. Plateaus are going to happen. Remember why you started and how far you've already come. Gratitude fuels determination. Then look forward to the next realistic goal you've set to keep hope alive.

Remember that high weight loss expectations lead to giving up. A 10% weight loss maintained is better for you than losing 100 pounds and gaining it all back.

When the weight refuses to come off, do not eat less. That is a common weight loss mistake. Instead of eating less, exercise more.

Are you already a type 2 diabetic? It doesn't matter. These tips will work for you too. Insulin and medications won't prevent you from reaching the milestones you are aiming for. Only one thing will stop you, and that is giving up.

I've learned this lesson at 62 years old even though I have

type 2 diabetes and take insulin every day. Go to my website's weight loss page and you'll see how much I've lost already.

Martha Zimmer invites you to visit her website and learn more about type 2 diabetes, its complications and how you can deal with them, as well as great tips for eating healthy that will make living with diabetes less painful.

PREDIABETES - HOW DO YOU KNOW IF YOU HAVE IT?

Prediabetes Defined or those people that have developed some form of diabetes, mostly those that have type 2 diabetes, they were most likely prediabetic and may not have even known it. As is the case with diabetes, it is the level of glucose in the blood that determines this condition. Usually the blood glucose levels are higher than normal but do not typically diagnosed as diabetes (again mostly type 2 diabetes). If you are thinking how can this be...if the medical profession is aware of this condition, why does it not get identified? Seems logical but in actuality it can be easily missed. In fact it is estimated by the American Diabetes Association that there are 79 million people in the US that go undiagnosed with this condition. Think of it this way, have you ever taken your car into the dealership for a noise only to get there and not hear the noise? I know that has happened to me on more than one occasion. Well it is similar to identifying a higher than normal blood glucose level. You may not have a higher level at the time you visit your doctor but did so just a couple days earlier and as a result it gets missed. One way to better detect if you are prediabetic is to monitor and record your own blood glucose levels at regular intervals. Provide this information to your medical professional for review. Remember early detection is the key here, especially if you have a family history of diabetes or are experiencing symptoms that could be attributed to diabetes. As the saying goes....no harm...no foul.

Prediabetes Symptoms, Health Implications??

Some of the symptoms that may indicate prediabetes are the following:

- ✓ Frequent infections of the gum, bladder or skin
- ✓ Feeling fatigued
- ✓ Impaired vision
- ✓ Constant or unusual thirst
- ✓ Loss of feeling in the hands/feet
- ✓ Frequent urination
- ✓ Bruises/cuts that heal slow

As we noted previously there is a greater chance of developing diabetes and in particular type 2 diabetes if you are prediabetic. Studies by the Diabetes Prevention Program indicated that every year 11% of the people with prediabetes developed type 2 diabetes during three years of follow-up. However there have been other studies that indicate that it could be as long as 10 years. It depends ultimately on what steps are taken to manage your blood glucose levels. This is supported by additional research that indicates that long term damage to the heart and circulatory system may occur with being prediabetic.

What is My Prediabetes Risk? Who should be Tested?

There are three main tests to determine if your metabolism is normal, pre-diabetic or diabetic.

- ✓ Fasting Plasma Glucose Test (FPG) - Fasting overnight w/ glucose testing prior to eating
- ✓ <100mg/dl (normal), =100mg/dl <126mg/dl (prediabetic), =126mg/dl (diabetic)

- ✓ AIC Test - average range of glucose over the past 3-4 months
- ✓ <5,7%(normal), =5.7% <6.5%(prediabetic), = 6.5%(diabetic)
- ✓ Oral Glucose Tolerance Test (OGTT) - Fasting overnight w/ testing first thing in the morning & 2 hours after consuming a glucose rich drink
- ✓ <140mg/dl(normal), =140mg/dl <200mg/dl(prediabetic), =200mg/dl(diabetic)

An important point to make here is that if an OGTT test reveals an abnormal blood glucose level you are considered to have impaired glucose tolerance (IGT). For an abnormal glucose level on a FGP test, you are considered to have impaired fasting glucose (IFG). While these may have different medical terms they both indicate the same condition prediabetes.

If you want to find out your risk level, check out the American Diabetes Association Website. There you can print out for free a Diabetes Self Test form that when filled out will give you a better idea if you need one of the previous tests mentioned. A high score may suggest that additional testing is necessary. Find out your score!

One final note on testing for prediabetes. While this condition occurs in all races and age groups, African Americans, Latinos, Asian Americans/Pacific Islanders and Native Americans are at a higher risk of developing this condition. However if you are 45 or older and overweight you should be checked at your next regular visit. If you are under the age of 45 but have high blood pressure, low HDL cholesterol and high triglycerides, a family history of gestational diabetes or diabetes, you should also be tested at your next checkup.

Prediabetes Confirmed Can it be Treated?

As we stated before, it depends on how the individual chooses to manage their blood glucose levels that determines any success of treatment. The good news is that prediabetes is not diabetes and does not have many of the medical impacts as diabetes. So the goal is to keep it that way and one of the best ways to that is make changes in diet and increase the amount of exercise. A study by the Diabetes Prevention Program (DPP) indicated that 30 minutes of moderate physical exercise and a reduction of 7% in body weight resulted in a 58% reduced risk to developing type 2 diabetes over medication alone.

Now if you are saying 7% reduction in body weight!!! Well there are many resources available on the Web that can help you lose much more than 7%. Look at this as an opportunity to finally get that slim figure you have been promising to get every New Years Eve resolution. Remember the steps you take now will greatly reduce the potential for developing Diabetes later. As always, seek the advice of your doctor before starting any exercise routine

HOW TO STOP PREDIABETES AND HIGH BLOOD SUGAR LEVELS DESTROYING YOUR HEALTH?

Prediabetes, well you would think you either have type 2 diabetes or you don't! In one way it's true, you don't yet have type 2 but it's certainly trying to catch you. Already changes are going on inside your body and they have been for a time now, probably a couple of years. These changes have affected how your body uses both insulin and sugar.

Blood sugar levels vary through the day, your levels are lower before eating and naturally higher following a meal. Your recent test for fasting blood sugars showing you were prediabetic, would have been between 100 to 125 mg/dl (5.5 to 6.9 mmol/l). Levels higher than 126 mg/dl (7 mmol/l) indicate full blown type 2 diabetes. The impaired or prediabetic range for the glucose tolerance test is between 140 to 199 mg/dl (7.8 to 11 mmol/l).

What does this mean to you?

it means your pancreas may not be making enough insulin

your pancreas is still making enough insulin but your body is not responding well to insulin's commands

the amount of insulin being produced, be it a normal amount or more, isn't enough to "open the doors" to certain body cells, and the cells have stopped responding to insulin's commands to let blood sugar in

you eat more food than your body can deal with

could be one or several of the above

What action should you take?

are you overweight or obese? What is your waist measurement ... 40 inches (100 cm) for a male or 34 inches (84 cm) for a female puts you in type 2 diabetes territory. Stabilize your weight then lower your weight to a healthy level. You will gain benefits from any weight loss. You could consult with a dietitian who specializes in diabetes or find a diet book that sets out a

style of eating that you will stick with. It needs to be a long-term plan, slow and steady

increase your physical activity. Keep it simple, maybe start walking. Start out small, ten minutes the first days and gradually increase the time up to 20 to 30 minutes four or five times a week. This helps with weight loss. But also with reducing your blood sugars; exercise uses glucose stored in your muscles which then signals your body to send along more from your bloodstream

if your health care provider prescribed medications you will need to follow his instructions. When you lose weight have your health care provider review your medications. Weight loss and major lifestyle changes may actually be more effective than intensive medications.

learn to monitor your blood sugar levels because that's how you will know straight away if you are keeping your blood sugar levels near to normal

Type 2 diabetes does not have to control your life. You can not only prevent disabling complications but effectively stop progression of this condition.

WHAT YOU NEED TO KNOW ABOUT PRE DIABETES SYMPTOMS

Most of the time, borderline diabetes or simply pre diabetes has no symptoms or signs. Acanthosis nigricans is a pre diabetes symptom characterized as the darkened areas of skin. This common sign affect the areas in the armpits, knuckles, elbows and the neck.

The following are some of the classic red flags of type 2 diabetes mellitus that you should watch out:

- ✓ Blurry vision
- ✓ frequent urination
- ✓ increased thirst
- ✓ fatigue

See a doctor if you are concerned about diabetes milletus or if you happen to notice a particular pre diabetes symptom or sign such as frequent urination, blurry vision, increased thirst and fatigue. Ask your doctor regarding blood glucose screening if you have any of the following risk factors for borderline diabetes:

- ✓ you are aged over 45 years old
- ✓ you are overweight, with a body mass index above 25
- ✓ you have a family history of type 2 diabetes
- ✓ you are currently inactive
- ✓ you have a high blood pressure
- ✓ you have polycystic ovary syndrome

✓ you are Hispanic, Asian-American, African-American, American Indian or a Pacific Islander
✓ you regularly sleep 5 and a half hours at night or even fewer
✓ your HDL or high-density lipoprotein cholesterol is below 35 mg/dL or triglyceride level is above 250 mg/dL
✓ when you were pregnant or gave birth to a baby who weighed more than 9 lbs, you have developed gestational diabetes

Early pre diabetes symptom although alarming, can also be misleading. Keep in mind that prevention is always better than cure. If you are currently exhibiting signs, it is a better idea to have them checked out. In doing so, it will either help you to change your lifestyle before a full blown diabetes mellitus takes hold or put your mind at rest.

5 SIGNS OF PRE DIABETES

Today millions of Americans are struggling with either Type 1 or Type 2 Diabetes. It has become an epidemic for Men, Women and Children. Fortunately it is one of the most studied diseases today.

What is PreDiabetes? It is when an individual has been seen by their Doctor and they have not been diagnosed with either Type 1 or 2 Diabetes, but their sugar/glucose count is hirer than it should be. At this point the Doctor sees no reason to recommend any medication but encourages them to change their lifestyle by eating healthier and exercising to deter the next phase of Diabetes.

This book really focus on those who have not been diagnosed with Diabetes, but may have one or more of the risk factors, such as:

- ✓ Obesity
- ✓ Age
- ✓ Family History of Diabetes
- ✓ Sedentary life style-do not lead an active life/no exercise
- ✓ Have Cancer
- ✓ Consumes a large sum of sugar in their daily diet
- ✓ Diet full of high fatty foods

There are actually signs that one can look for so they are not totally caught off guard when they begin to have some health issues.

1. Energy Level - Feel tired and sluggish most of the time, especially after eating a meal.

2. Physical appearance - Body changing. Increasing weight around the waistline, mid section, belly, hips, buttocks, etc.

3. Physical issues - May experience frequent heart burn, frequent urination and dry mouth.

4. Medical issues - Glucose elevated above 90mg/dl, high cholesterol and high triglycerides.

5. Eating Clues - Always hungry. Craves certain foods, especially simple carbohydrates (cookies, cakes, pies, chips, etc.). Just can't seem to get full. Desires to drink a lot of pops/sodas and other high sugary beverages.

If these signs become evident to you make an appointment and see your family Doctor.

By being proactive you can decrease your chances of becoming Diabetic and live a long and healthier life .

YOU CAN PROACTIVELY DEFEAT PREDIABETES

Prediabetes is a wakeup call that alerts you that your blood sugar has crossed the redline line of normality requiring you to take some action or it will lead to full diabetes. Diabetes is a disease that causes the body to not be able to make enough insulin. This lack of insulin then makes the glucose levels above what's considered normal. Diabetes is a progressive disease that can cause many complications if it's not adequately managed.

However, long before full blown diabetes manifests, there is a period of time where type 2 diabetes can be prevented. During the stage where there's a higher risk of prediabetes, by being proactive with your health, you can stop it dead in its tracks.

To understand prediabetes then we must ask, "Who Is at Risk for Prediabetes?" While it is possible that prediabetes can happen to anyone, there are several risk factors that one needs to have that can raise the threshold of the level of risk. Learning these risks enables one to take steps to eliminate as many of these factors as possible.

One of the most common risk factors for developing prediabetes is carrying a lot of weight specifically around the abdomen (belly fat). Women with waist size of 35 inches or greater, have a high risk level of prediabetes. Men who have abdomens that are 40 inches or greater are at a higher risk.

The heavier that a person is, the more fat that person will

carry. Carrying excess fat makes it more difficult for the cells to use insulin the proper way.

When this happens, you enter a stage called insulin resistance because the cells are resisting insulin uptake from the blood. This stage causes the blood sugar levels to increase.

Lack of some form of regular exercise is also a common factor in developing prediabetes. A sedentary lifestyle can lead to making your cells insulin resistant. This is what makes exercise one of the top to do items that can help prevent prediabetes from happening. Regular activity helps to

maintain a healthier body weight, in addition to helping the body burn glucose. In these ways, exercise helps the body not to be insulin resistant.

Prediabetes can happen to anyone at any time. But one of the big risk factors is getting older. Once you hit middle age, your risk factor goes up. Some studies point to the possibility that this risk increases simply because people tend to be less focused on maintaining a healthy lifestyle.

When it comes to prediabetes, you can't escape how your genetics play into it. If there's a family history of diabetes, then your risk of developing prediabetes is significantly higher than people with no history of diabetes.

There are certain life issues peculiar to women that can arise that can also raise the risk level. Women who had gestational diabetes, and their glucose levels went back to the normal range after the pregnancy ended, are at a higher risk of getting diagnosed with prediabetes later in life. Another issue polycystic ovary syndrome (PCOS). This condition causes the estrogen and progesterone levels to become out of balance. The condition is linked with weight gain, obesity, and diabetes, raising the risk of prediabetes.

This may be a surprise for some to learn but having trouble sleeping has also been linked to prediabetes. When you don't get the right amount of sleep, it can cause your cells to develop insulin resistance. It's the insulin resistance that causes the prediabetes to happen. Those at risk include people who struggle with insomnia, those who work night shifts, third shifts or whose sleep is often interrupted.

DIABETIC MEAL PLAN - TAKE CONTROL OF YOUR DIABETES TODAY

Those who are find themselves experiencing diabetic and prediabetic symptoms now have available free diabetic diet meal plans. If your diet is not controlled, diabetes can become a life threatening disease as soon as a matter of months. When there are free diabetic plans being released for all those who have diabetes, there is no reason you can not gain control of the disease.

Practically every weight-loss program is based upon diabetic diet lists.

Medication available for diabetes today aids in maintaining insulin levels. All the medication available, however, pales in comparison to the effectiveness of a properly planned meal plan. The medical community needs patients to be more dependent upon them, so they are willing to put your health at risk to hide the importance of a properly planned diet. Take control of your diabetes with the proper proportion of carbohydrates, protein and fat. If you are overweight, limit your caloric intake. There are diets available that have 1200 - 1500 and even 1800 calories so you can receive the nutrients that your body requires and you will not be hungry.

In order to control diabetic symptoms - current diabetic meal plans must be correctly and professionally prepared. There have been several clients, whom after following the strict diet plan with exercise, came off most of their medications and lost a significant amount of body fat.

If you're experiencing these symptoms of diabetes, do yourself a favor and conquer this disease by getting information on these free diet plans.

Only with diet, not medication, can fully prevent and reverse the onset of diabetes type II

HOW TO PREVENT DIABETES WITH A PRE-DIABETIC DIET

There are many people around the globe who suffer from the same diseases that we all know as diabetes. As we talk about diabetes, it is very difficult to know whether a person is affected by the disease because no symptoms of diabetes in the early stages. In many cases a lot of people with the type 2 diabetes even before they were diagnosed for the pre-diabetic condition. This is a condition where the level of blood glucose is high but not high enough that the doctor can diagnose a person with diabetes. According to recent studies, results showed that there are many people and continues to grow, with pre-diabetes.

The basic thing that you need to understand about the diabetes is, that it is a diseases that will highly affect the production of insulin in the human body. Insulin is the hormones that are needed to convert all the sugar and starch, that we consume, into the energy that we need in our daily life. Once the production of these hormones is affected, they are unable to convert the sugar into energy, hence increasing the glucose level in the human body.

Contrary to popular misconception, because we talk about pre-diabetes is curable in such a way that not only can be cured, but it stop the growth of type 2 diabetes. All you need to make sure you ask your doctor to keep track of your level of glucose in the blood so that in cases where there are signs of pre-diabetes, you can take certain measures. The best is that you must follow a diet and exercise plan. This gives you only a delay, or it may also help prevent type 2 diabetes. In addition, you will see a big difference in pre-diabetes that affects them.

You do not need a doctor of all time, as there is a great deal to be done to avert the progress of type 2 diabetes and get free of pre-diabetes that affects them. The American Diabetes Association has a prosperity of resources for citizens with diabetes. All of us need to understand the fact that if anyone is pre-diabetic around us, all we need to do is to make sure that we give them some proper physical workout tips and give them some proper diet that will help them in getting rid of the pre-diabetic condition and it will also prevent the further growth of the type 2 diabetes in the patient.

PREDIABETES - AN AUTHENTIC DIAGNOSIS THAT IS MORE THAN GLUCOSE INTOLERANCE

Prediabetes is a real disorder of personal metabolism and a true disease. Prediabetes exists as a condition when one's fasting blood glucose level ranges 100-125 mg/dl or when one's random hemoglobin A1c value ranges 5.8-6.4. Normal fasting glucose is less than 99 mg/dl but greater than 70 mg/dl, and normal hemoglobin A1c values are 5.7 or less.

Prediabetes is recognized and so-named because nearly 50% of affected individuals will progress to overt Diabetes Mellitus over 5 years. And, in repeated public health surveys and studies, prediabetes is associated with accelerated atherosclerosis, coronary artery disease, and progressive kidney function impairment first manifest by protein leakage into the urine.

Glucose is a simple sugar that our body uses for energy. Table sugar is called sucrose, and sucrose is broken down to glucose in our intestine after eating. Glucose is then absorbed into our blood and travels to all of our tissues, where it is transported into tissue cells by the action of insulin. Our bodies are set so that glucose in our blood stream is transported into tissue cells within a prompt time frame of less than 2 hours. If this process is not working normally, then glucose will circulate at higher than normal blood values and this leads to biological trouble.

A normal blood glucose level after no food for 8 hours (fasting glucose) is between 70 and 99 mg/dL. A normal blood glucose level two hours after eating is less than 140 mg/dL. The glucose surge into our blood stream triggers insulin release from our pancreas. The quantity of insulin released is set by quantity of glucose sensed by our pancreas and sensitivity of insulin action in our organs. Insulin drives glucose uptake into our tissue cells.

Diabetes mellitus exists when:

Two consecutive fasting blood glucose tests are equal to or greater than 126 mg/dl -- or,

A random non-fasting blood glucose value is greater than 200 mg/dl -- or,

A hemoglobin A1c test is equal to or greater than 6.5 percent.

Prediabetes exists as a real medical condition that requires specific interventions when

A fasting blood glucose value is between 100-125 mg/dL, or,

A hemoglobin A1c value is between 5.7 - 6.4 percent, or,

A random blood glucose value is between 140 mg/dL and 199 mg/d.

Prediabetes is tissue glucose intolerance and is an impairment of glucose utilization,and it truly does lead to health changes and organ alterations that doctors call complications. It leads to overt diabetes mellitus in over

50% of persons.

Thus, prediabetes is designated as a true medical condition that requires actions - adjustment in diet, adjustment in activity, weight loss, and often medication. No longer can "glucose intolerance" be simply mentioned and not registered as an authentic medical problem.

If you have been told that you have glucose intolerance, realize that you have a disease of your glucose metabolism that causes trouble to you. Ask for more information. Your doctor should provide a care plan to you and track your condition as any other disease or medical problem is tracked. More about this shall be explained in subsequent articles.

Rex Mahnensmith, M.D. is a Board Certified Internal Medicine Physician with special interests in metabolic disorders. He has served as full time Clinician Educator at 3 medical schools over 27 years. He now serves in a Community Health Clinic as primary care physician. He is most interested in helping individuals be well by preventing disease and managing evolving disease so that complications do not arise. This article commences a series that will inform and serve as a guide to wellness for individuals with metabolic disorders.

HOW TO FIND OUT IF YOU HAVE PREDIABETES

How does prediabetes differ from Type 1 or Type 2 diabetes?

Understanding the production of insulin is the first step to understanding diabtes. Insulin is a hormone that helps your cells metabolize glucose or sugar found in the foods that you eat. If you suffer from diabetes, your body fails to produce the right insulin level. Therefore, the amount of insulin in your body may be too little or too much, which can lead to serious medical conditions. A build-up of glucose in your blood, for instance, can result in damages to the blood vessels in your heart, kidneys, and nervous system.

Individuals who suffer from prediabetes have high glucose levels, although they're rarely as high as those in diabetic patients. And even though those with prediabetes may not present obvious symptoms, they still be at risk of heart ailments due to poor diet or exercise habits. When you suffer from this condition, your pancreas may be unable to produce the right amount of insulin after each meal, and this affects the clearing of the incoming glucose from your blood. Another effect of pre diabetes is insulin resistance, which prevents glucose from being carried to your bloodstream efficiently. Moreover, pre diabetes can eventually result in type 2 diabetes, as well as other medical concerns such as stroke and heart ailments. People who are prediabetic may also have a huge chance of developing these conditions, as compared to individuals who have never suffered from pre diabetes.

Keep in mind that you may have prediabetes without showing any outward symptoms. While you might think the lack of symptoms is an indication that you should not take this seriously, you would be wrong. Prediabetes symptoms can be easily managed with diet and exercise to prevent them from turning into Type 2 diabetes. Maybe you are feeling a little more tired than usual. You might be thirsty more often and going to the bathroom more often. Some people with prediabetes experience these symptoms and attribute them to something else, like being overworked. The only way to know for sure is to check your blood sugar level with diabetic supplies.

Plan to check your blood sugar level in the morning, before you've even had a drink of water or cup of coffee. Have your supplies ready. Keep in mind that your glucometer and test strips are sensitive to temperatures, so they need to be kept in the area you will be using them for a more accurate reading. Test your sugar as soon as you get out of bed. Before eating in the morning your blood sugar should be between 70 and 100. A reading of between 101 and 126 is one recognized indicator of prediabtes.. If your blood sugar is above 126, this is an indication of diabetes.After eating, wait two hours and check your sugar again. Two hours after eating, your blood sugar should be between 70 and 140. If it is between 141 and 200, this is a sign of prediabetes. If it is above 200, it is a sign of diabetes. Continue to monitor your blood sugar to determine if you show symptoms or prediabetes or full blown diabetes.

Fortunately, you can do something to improve your condition and prevent Type 1 or Type 2 diabetes. By adopting a healthier lifestyle that includes regular exercise, a wholesome diet and weight maintenance, you maintain your health and help prevent future conditions.

HOW TO STOP PREDIABETES IN ITS TRACKS

According to the CDC, 9.3% of the population has diabetes, BUT, 3X as many people have prediabetes. Essentially, 1 out of 3 individuals have prediabetes, but the sad part is that 90% of them don't even know it! Today, we are shining light on this condition and what you can do to drastically reduce your odds of getting diabetes.

Sugar often takes the brunt of the blame when it comes to the onset of diabetes, but there are many lifestyle factors that all contribute to the development (and prevention) of diabetes. Staying on top of your health and getting proactive can help you stop it for good.

Fellow Registered Dietitian, Jill Weisenberger, is a Certified Diabetes Educator, Health Coach and author of the newest American Diabetes Association book, Prediabetes: A Complete Guide. This book is "Your Lifestyle Reset to Stop Prediabetes and Other Chronic Illnesses."

An expert in all things diabetes, Jill makes the nutrition science understandable, practical and delicious. As a mom and wife, she knows the real-life struggles of feeding a family and making health a priority among the ins and outs of a busy life. Answering some of the most common questions about prediabetes, she is clearing up confusion about carbs, medications, symptoms, genetics and MORE in my interview with her.

Whether you have a family history of diabetes, have recently been told you have prediabetes or simply want to stay proactive managing your health,

Being diagnosed with prediabetes doesn't mean you will develop diabetes. Your doctor can help you come up with an effective plan to keep your blood sugar low, so that you can keep diabetes away for good.

Prediabetes, the common precursor to diabetes, affects more than 86 million Americans, according to the Centers for Disease Control and Prevention. An estimated 90 percent of people with prediabetes don't even realize they have this condition. Experts also estimate that three out of four people with prediabetes will eventually develop diabetes.

The good news, however, is that once your doctor determines that your blood sugar is high enough to be classified as prediabetes (but not high enough to be diabetes), there are plenty of preventive measures you can take to stop the onset of full diabetes. The window of opportunity to prevent or slow the progression of prediabetes to type 2 diabetes is about three to six years.

Make sure you take the following steps to be on the right path to fight prediabetes and take the appropriate steps to lower your blood sugar level.

1. Take the quiz

One of the first things you can do to find out if you are at risk for prediabetes or type 2 diabetes, is take the American Diabetes Association's Risk Test. The ADA offers a helpful one-minute quiz, which features questions about age, weight and your family history of diabetes. The results will determine if you are at a low, moderate or high risk of diabetes.

2. Check your glucose level

If your quiz results determine that you have a high chance of developing diabetes, be sure to consult with your doctor and ask for a glucose test to check your blood's sugar level.

3. Reduce calorie and fat intake

Research has shown that losing 5 to 7 percent of your body weight can help decrease blood glucose levels and help other health goals, such as improving blood pressure, raising HDL (good cholesterol) and lowering triglycerides. You can accomplish this goal by consuming fruits, vegetables and whole grains and staying away from processed foods. Nutritionists often recommend sticking with a variety of food, so that your taste buds won't get bored and you can continue a healthy diet.

4. Stay active

Try to hit 150 minutes of physical activity, or only half-hour a day for five days, in one week. You can achieve many of your health goals by keeping

your mind and body trained. Recommended exercises include walking, jogging, running, biking, swimming or group exercises, such as yoga or spinning.

5. Keep monitoring your blood glucose level

The ADA recommends that people who are diagnosed with

prediabetes get their glucose levels checked annually. You may even ask your health care provider whether you need a home glucose monitor to check the state of your prediabetes. That's because the possibility of recurrence always exists. Aging, gaining weight or falling back on habits, such as smoking, overeating or not exercising can cause blood glucose levels to rise again.

6. You may need medication

If you are at high risk of developing diabetes, your doctor may recommend medication to help you manage it. Medications to control cholesterol and high blood pressure may also be prescribed.

Nearly 20 million Americans are headed down the road to diabetes, but modest weight loss and a bit more activity would be enough to turn them around. These people have prediabetes, meaning their above-normal blood sugar levels signal a high risk of developing type 2 diabetes within the next 10 years.

More women opting for preventive mastectomy - but should they be?

Rates of women who are opting for preventive mastectomies, such as Angeline Jolie, have increased by an estimated 50 percent in recent years, experts say. But many doctors are puzzled because the operation doesn't carry a 100 percent guarantee, it's major surgery and women have other options, from a once-a-day pill to careful monitoring.

What stresses moms most? Themselves, survey says

A combination of obesity, inactivity and genetics is responsible. But most people with prediabetes aren't aware they have it, and insurers may not cover testing for or treatment of the condition.

"It's really quite a remarkable opportunity, but it's not as if everyone is rushing to be identified," says Dr. Daniel Einhorn of the Scripps Whittier Institute for Diabetes in La Jolla, Calif. Many people may be reluctant to get tested and labeled especially if they're feeling fine, he adds. But catching the condition before it turns into full-blown diabetes can be a lifesaver.

People with Type 2 diabetes either lose the ability to respond to insulin, or their bodies no longer make enough of the hormone. Insulin helps the body use glucose as fuel, so without it sugar builds up in the bloodstream. Over time, especially if blood sugar levels are not kept in check, diabetes can boost a person's risk of heart disease and cause damage to the eyes, kidneys, nerves and other body tissues.

Prediabetes used to be called impaired fasting glucose, but federal officials and diabetes experts introduced the new name last year. The term is not only more consumer-friendly, but does more to convey the urgency of the condition, says Dr. Gene Barrett, president of the American Diabetes Association.

Prediabetes is like the warning light in your car that clicks on when you're about to run out of gas, says Roberta Anding, a registered dietitian and certified diabetes educator at Texas Children's Hospital in Houston. There's danger ahead, she explains, but it's in your power to do something about it.

Weight loss and exercise help

Weight loss and exercise really will help, experts say, and there's no need to pare off every extra pound or undertake an elaborate, strenuous exercise program. The Diabetes Prevention Program study found that people with prediabetes who walked or did other exercise for a half-hour at least five times a week and lost 5 to 7 percent of their total weight cut their risk of developing full-fledged diabetes by nearly 60 percent. The lifestyle changes were twice as effective as taking a pill.

While people in this study got extensive support for their efforts, including one-on-one counseling and intensive follow-up, other trials in which patients got less intense support have had similarly good results, notes Barrett. "There are lots of ways to do it without quite all those bells and whistles," he adds.

What can really help people stay motivated, Barrett says, is periodic contact with a health professional like a nutritionist or nurse even just a five-minute phone call every week or two. Many institutions and hospitals have programs that offer such interventions, but patients themselves will likely have to foot at least some of the bill.

Get screened

People with prediabetes belong a larger group of individuals with a condition known as insulin resistance syndrome (IRS), in which the body gradually loses sensitivity to the key blood-sugar-regulating hormone.

Individuals with IRS tend to have a family history of heart

disease and diabetes, as well as a characteristic type of obesity in which weight settles around the abdomen rather than below the waist, high levels of triglycerides in the blood, high blood pressure, and low levels of "good" HDL cholesterol. They are also at risk of heart disease and may face a greater chance of developing certain cancers.

While most people with IRS have normal blood sugar levels, roughly 20 percent have levels that climb out of the normal range, and are considered to have prediabetes.

The ADA recommends doctors screen everyone 45 and older for prediabetes, particularly obese people, and that those with certain risk factors be tested earlier.

In late October, the ADA broadened its definition of prediabetes to include people with fasting blood glucose levels of 100 milligrams per deciliter (mg/dL) of blood. Previously, the cutoff point had been 110 mg/dL. This shift increased the population of prediabetics by 20 percent.There's no one quick test to identify prediabetes. Instead doctors look at several different factors before making the diagnosis.

Educate yourself

If you are diagnosed with prediabetes, what should you do? "See your doctor a couple of times a year," Einhorn says. "Meet with a registered dietitian, an exercise physiologist, learn how to become fit, to eat thoughtfully."

While insurance coverage for prediabetes care is lacking, Einhorn notes, some nutrition programs may be partially covered or offered at a nominal fee.

The ADA can help you find certified diabetes educators, support groups and diabetes education programs in your neighborhood.

People with prediabetes may also benefit from certain medications, including baby aspirin and niacin, the diabetes drug metformin, and mild blood pressure medications such as ACE inhibitors and angiotensin receptor blockers.

Eric Goodis is living proof that diabetes can be beat with weight loss and exercise. Diagnosed in 2001, when he was 140 pounds overweight and sedentary, the San Diego record-label owner went on diabetes medication and started watching his diet and exercising more. Within six months he no longer needed the medication and was able to get off the drugs he'd also been taking for high blood pressure and high cholesterol. He managed to lose all his excess weight in 11 months, and is now, at 52, an avid cyclist logging 200 miles a week with no signs of diabetes.

Goodis began his exercise program very slowly because he had to. "It was almost strolling and it was the best I could do," he remembers. He took two walks a day, and on each walk would push himself to pass one more house before he turned around. And as he became more active and the weight came off, it got easier to follow his diet.

"The first thing I would tell people is 'don't panic, it's manageable,'" Goodis said. "It is manageable if you take it piece-by-piece, hour-by-hour, day-by-day. It's almost kind of like those 12-step programs."

Other advice? Get educated about diabetes, work closely with your doctor, don't be addicted to the scale and don't get discouraged, Goodis says. "It's not a steady road to improvement," he explains. "You kind of have up days and down days."

Goodis gave himself a year to lose the weight, and advises others to give themselves a similarly generous time frame. "It goes a lot quicker than you think."

DIABETES SHOPPING LIST
Fruit

You'll need 2 to 4 servings of fresh or frozen fruit a day. While in the store, you can use an apple to approximate a serving of fruit. Try not to plan out ahead of time what fruit you will buy; sometimes, for one reason or another, fruit just doesn't look good. Many fruits can be substituted for each other in recipes anyway. Instead, plan for how many servings of fruit you'll need to buy. And when you're in the store, buy what is fresh, seasonal, and/or on sale.

Meat, Fish, And Protein-Rich Food

You'll need 2 to 3 servings of lean protein-rich foods a day. Visualize a deck of cards to help approximate a 3 ounce serving of meat or fish. One egg or 1/2 cup of tofu is also a serving of meat. Skinless chicken and/or turkey, fish, lean cuts of beef, pork, eggs or egg substitute, and low-fat peanut butter should be on your list.

Non-Starchy Vegetables

Half of your lunch and dinner plate should be vegetables, and vegetables are also handy to have on hand for diabetes-friendly snacks. So plan on buying enough fresh or frozen vegetables to meet those needs. Same as with fruit, try to plan out how much you'll need, but wait until you get to the store to see what looks like the best buy. That being said, dark green vegetables like spinach, dark lettuce, and broccoli as well as yellow-orange vegetables, like sweet peppers and carrots typically have the highest vitamin and mineral content. Avocados are technically a fruit but are often used more like a vegetable in recipes. They are packed with healthy fats and are useful in rounding out a diabetes-friendly meal. Onions and garlic are both low glycemic foods rich in antioxidant nutrients. They are useful for adding flavor while keeping cooking low in fat and should be on your list.

Fat

Monounsaturated and polyunsaturated oils such as olive, canola, corn, sunflower, or soybean oils should be on your list. Also, look for lower fat butter-flavored spreads made with these oils (to use in place of butter on bread), and fat-free cooking spray to use in sautéing and baking.

Nuts, Beans

Almonds and walnuts are great for topping salads or even mixing in cereal or yogurt. Canned black beans, kidney beans, garbanzo beans, or really any variety of legume should be on your list. Canned beans should be rinsed well before use, to remove excess sodium, but are quick to cook and very useful in diabetes meal plans.

Low-Fat Dairy

Plan for 2 to 3 servings a day of nonfat or low-fat milk or yogurt (1 cup = serving), or low-fat cottage cheese (1/4 cup serving).

Whole Grains, Starchy Vegetables, And Lentils

Ignore the labels that say, "this product contains X grams of whole grains per serving." Instead, flip products over and look at their nutrition labels. Choose the ones that are highest in fiber. Brown rice, whole-wheat pasta, high-fiber cereals, and high-fiber bread should be on your list. Alternate grains like quinoa, barley, and bulgur can often be substituted for rice in recipes. Sweet potatoes, corn, sweet peas, butternut squash, and lentils can also replace grains in a diabetes meal plan.

"Diabetic" Products

You may want to consider putting an alternative sweetener on your grocery list to use in place of real sugar in coffee, tea, and recipes. Zero-calorie beverages like freshly brewed iced tea, diet sodas, and fruit-flavored waters could go on your list to give you some drink options that won't affect your blood sugar. And since everyone needs an occasional treat, look for a low-sugar cookie or cake just remember that it is actually the total carbohydrate in a product (not sugar) that will affect your blood sugar.

CONCLUSION

Lastly, even though age above 40 years, male gender, higher BMI, high WHR, and systolic BP above 140 mm Hg were at higher risk of being prediabetes, statistically significant association was found only for age and systolic BP. Whereas statistically significant association was found for age, sex, BMI, WHR, diastolic BP, and systolic BP with diabetes. Shamima Akter et al. reported significant and positive association for prediabetes with older age and high body weight among Bangladesh adults.

Diabetes is preceded by impaired fasting glucose (IFG) resulting in a pre-diabetic state which can exist undetected for many years, causing irreversible damage to vital organs. Pre-diabetes is a practical term referring to Impaired Fasting Glucose (IFG), impaired glucose tolerance or a glycosylated hemoglobin (A1c) of 6.0% to 6.4%, each of which places individuals at high risk of developing diabetes and it complications. The World Health Organization criteria for diagnosing pre-diabetes are fasting plasma glucose level of between 6.1 mmol/l to 6.9 mmol/l. A fasting plasma glucose level 7.0 mmol/l or more meets the criteria for the diagnosis of diabetes. Fasting value for venous and capillary plasma glucose are identical

Mohammed et al. reported statistically significant association with male gender, age above 45 years, and higher than average BMI.Mohan et al. showed obesity, abdominal obesity, and hypertension to be significantly associated with incident diabetes. Anjana et al. reported significant risk factors for prediabetes to be age, abdominal obesity, and hypertension.

Joji Ishikawa et al. reported that prediabetes was associated with masked hypertension. Pramono and Pradana Soewondo reported sex, age, socioeconomic status, education level, obesity, central obesity, hypertension, and no smoking habit as predictive factors for prediabetes. In our study, smoking habits were associated with diabetes but not for prediabetes. Mihardja et al. reported smoking habit as determinant factors on prediabetes/diabetes. In our study, alcohol consumption increased risk of prediabetes and diabetes. Similar finding was reported by Cullmann et al. that total alcohol consumption and binge drinking increased the risk of prediabetes and Type 2 diabetes in men. Ghorpade et al. reported significant association with sex, age group, educational status, per capita income, family history of T2DM, overweight/obesity, and alcohol use.

Shweta Sahai et al. reported that IFG increased with increasing waist circumference and showed a significant correlation with increasing WHR. In our study, a negative association was found between physical activity and prediabetes and positive association for diabetes but it was not statistically significant. Farni et al. reported a negative association between measures of physical activity and the prevalence of prediabetes in middle

aged USA adults. In our study, the proportion of prediabetic and diabetic having two or more risk factors were higher compared to normal individuals. Similar clustering of risk factors among prediabetic and diabetic was reported by other authors. As the study was carried out among health seekers in a fixed mobile clinic and the proportion of female attendance out number male, the results cannot be extrapolated to the larger population.

Diabetes mellitus is chronic non-communicable disease associated with long term complications to the brain, kidney, and the heart. There is destruction and loss of the cells of the pancreas causing insulin deficiency; it may also result from abnormalities arising from resistance to insulin. Symptoms of hyperglycemia include polydipsia, polyphagia polyuria, blurred vision, weight loss, generalized pruritus, neuropathy, retinopathy, etc. Life threatening consequences of uncontrolled diabetes include diabetes-ketoacidosis, lactic acidosis and hyper-osmolar non-ketotic state

PREDIABETES DIET PLAN

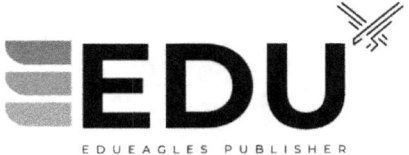

EDUEAGLES PUBLISHER